EUGENICAL STERILIZATION

This is a volume in the Arno Press collection

HISTORICAL ISSUES IN MENTAL HEALTH

See last pages of this volume for a complete list of titles

EUGENICAL STERILIZATION

THE COMMITTEE OF THE AMERICAN NEUROLOGICAL ASSOCIATION FOR THE INVESTIGATION OF EUGENICAL STERILIZATION:

ABRAHAM MYERSON, M.D.
JAMES B. AYER, M.D.
TRACY J. PUTNAM, M.D.
CLYDE E. KEELER, Sc.D.
LEO ALEXANDER, M.D.

ARNO PRESS
A New York Times Company
New York • 1980

Editorial Supervision: Brian Quinn

Reprint Edition 1980 by Arno Press Inc.

Reprinted from a copy in the Newark Public Library

HISTORICAL ISSUES IN MENTAL HEALTH
ISBN for complete set: 0-405-11900-3
See last pages of this volume for titles.

Manufactured in the United States of America

Library of Congress Cataloging in Publication Data

American Neurological Association. Committee for the
Investigation of Eugenical Sterilization.
Eugenical sterilization.

(Historical issues in mental health)
Reprint of the ed. published by Wright & Potter Print.
Co., Boston.
Bibliography: p.
Includes index.
1. Sterilization of criminals and defectives.
2. Eugenics. 3. Insanity. I. Myerson, Abraham,
1881-1948. II. Title. III. Series.
HV4989.A5 1979 362.2 78-22556
ISBN 0-405-11910-0

EUGENICAL STERILIZATION

THE MACMILLAN COMPANY
NEW YORK · BOSTON · CHICAGO · DALLAS
ATLANTA · SAN FRANCISCO

MACMILLAN & CO., Limited
LONDON · BOMBAY · CALCUTTA
MELBOURNE

THE MACMILLAN COMPANY
OF CANADA, Limited
TORONTO

EUGENICAL STERILIZATION

A Reorientation of the Problem

By

THE COMMITTEE OF THE AMERICAN NEUROLOGICAL ASSOCIATION FOR THE INVESTIGATION OF EUGENICAL STERILIZATION:

ABRAHAM MYERSON, M.D.
JAMES B. AYER, M.D.
TRACY J. PUTNAM, M.D.
CLYDE E. KEELER, Sc.D.
LEO ALEXANDER, M.D.

NEW YORK
THE MACMILLAN COMPANY
1936

Set up and printed. Published October, 1936.

PRINTED IN THE UNITED STATES OF AMERICA
BY THE STRATFORD PRESS, INC., NEW YORK

Dedicated to DR. ISRAEL STRAUSS, *former President of the American Neurological Association, without whose generous interest and persistent effort this book could not have appeared.*

FOREWORD

THE study and report of which this book is the result were carried on by a special committee appointed by the American Neurological Association.

The report was presented to and approved by the American Neurological Association at its annual meeting in 1935. It had such an enthusiastic reception that it was felt advisable to publish it in a more permanent form and make it available to the general public.

Both the study and the publication were made possible by a grant of money given by the Carnegie Foundation to the New York Academy of Medicine for the general purposes of a study of legal medicine. At the request of the Academy, the Carnegie Foundation agreed that a portion of this grant should be used for this specific purpose. The committee therefore desires to express its sincere appreciation to both the New York Academy of Medicine and the Carnegie Foundation.

STATEMENT OF THE COMMITTEE

THIS committee was appointed in May of 1934 by the American Neurological Association and its work was subsidized by a grant from the Carnegie Foundation. This grant made it possible for a more complete study to be made than would otherwise have been feasible. A preliminary report was published for circulation within the Association and read in June, 1935. It was accepted by the Association which has authorized its presentation here in an amplified form.

The committee has attempted to evaluate in a critical manner both the facts and the theories which constitute the subject-matter of the inheritance of the mental diseases, feeblemindedness, epilepsy, and crime. To survey the entire literature would be of no importance except from a historical point of view; to summon witnesses to give their impressions and opinions concerning the subject-matter of the study would be futile since whatever is pertinent and relevant has appeared in the literature.

In making recommendations we have endeavored to keep in mind the political and social complexion of America, since it is in that milieu that whatever laws are enacted must operate. We have tried to free our minds from the obsessive traditions of psychiatry and eugenics, and this report is, we believe, as unbiased and critical and as nearly objective as we could make it. We hope that the subject-matter of the report and the recommendations will be of value, both in evaluating past work and as the basis for legislative and, especially, for research activity.

ABRAHAM MYERSON, M. D. *Chairman*
JAMES B. AYER, M. D.
TRACY J. PUTNAM, M. D.
CLYDE E. KEELER, SC.D.,
Consultant in Genetics.
LEO ALEXANDER, M. D.,
Research Associate.

Boston, Massachusetts
June, 1936.

CONTENTS

Page

FOREWORD vii

STATEMENT OF THE COMMITTEE ix

I. INTRODUCTION 1

II. THE LAWS 7

III. MAIN ARGUMENTS FOR STERILIZATION 24

1. Analysis of Commitment Rate in Massachusetts and New York 28

2. Commitment Rate in Foreign Countries 36

3. Vital Statistics of the Mentally Defective and the Insane 40

IV. POINTS OF VIEW REGARDING STERILIZATION . . 59

V. GENETICS AND ITS RELATION TO EUGENICS . . 69

VI. STUDIES ON THE INHERITANCE OF MENTAL DISEASES 81

1. Polymorphism 82

2. Studies on Specific Mental Diseases 89

a. Schizophrenia 90

b. Manic-depressive Psychosis 107

c. Feeblemindedness 112

d. Epilepsy 136

VII. CHRONIC PROGRESSIVE NEUROLOGICAL DISEASES 145

VIII. CRIME 150

IX. TWINS 153

X. GENIUS AND EUGENICS 170

XI. RECOMMENDATIONS OF THE COMMITTEE . . . 177

XII. REFERENCES 184

INDEX 205

I

INTRODUCTION

The most primitive form of sterilization is undoubtedly castration. The impulse to inflict injury upon an enemy's genitalia as a measure of punishment and insult is a deeply rooted one in the human race, which finds expression at times among the most civilized modern nations, as well as among savages. When Heloise's uncle castrated Abélard, it was certainly with no eugenic purpose in mind, but to punish and show contempt for the man who had betrayed the honor of her family. There have been famous cases in the history of every community when such revenge has been taken, occasionally on a wholesale scale. The suspicion of a sadistic motive must always arise when genitalectomy is advocated for any group of physically healthy people, as for example, in Turkey and in occasional communities of the Western world where castration of certain classes of criminals has been prescribed by law.

Castration has also been practiced in the past for what might be termed commercial purposes. Thus, eunuchs were produced to act as safe servants and guardians in harems. Within modern times, juvenile tenor voices have been preserved by castration.

There has manifestly been a marked change in public opinion during the past century, and a growing appreciation of human rights—incomplete and inconsistent as it still is—has checked the employment of castration as an aggressive measure. The nineteenth century was one of humanitarian trend, of protest against oppression, and, on the whole, of progress toward democracy.

There have, however, been counter-currents. The thesis of Darwin that evolution takes place through survival of the fittest has often been interpreted to mean that any agency which interferes with "natural selection" works against the improvement of the race. The logical basis for this conclusion may be questioned: if "fitness" and "survival" are defined in terms of one another, broadening the basis of survival might be expected to broaden the conception of fitness. Some traits may have acquired a greater survival value in modern city life than they possessed in the jungle. On the other hand, it is not difficult to understand the uneasy feeling which many stern-minded people experience in contemplating the ameliorative social measures which permit the sick, the weak, and the unfortunate to survive and propagate. Many an eloquent voice has been raised against the pollution of the race which might be feared as a result.

The term "eugenics" originated with Galton, who based his social doctrines upon what was then known of heredity, a field of study in which he was a pioneer. Enormous strides have since been made in the field of genetics. It may, however, be seriously questioned whether many of the eugenic proposals now current take into account the newer genetic data; and further, whether the data upon which some are based—derived from experiments upon plants and lower animals—are applicable also to man.

We propose to examine certain fundamental questions which are involved directly or indirectly with the problem of sterilization. We shall begin with definitions. We shall then make some inquiry into the composition and background of some of the groups which have taken sides for or against a program of sterilization, for it must be realized that unrecognized prejudices and accidents of social status —what Calverton calls "cultural compulsives"—may be expected to color judgment in a controversy involving such fundamental issues. We shall abstract and summarize the various statutes now in force in different states in this country and abroad, and give brief statistics in regard to their enforcement.

We then propose to survey briefly the field of genetic knowledge, accepting without reserve the theory of the gene. We shall, however, also discuss the newer experiments which relate to the interplay of the environment with the genetic substance. We shall consider the experiments—not wholly conclusive, perhaps—which indicate that the germplasm may be injured by environmental forces and remain in an inferior or disorganized state for generations—experiments which raise the question whether what Forel has called "blastophoria" plays a part in the heredity of mental diseases and of feeblemindedness. We shall cite the opinions of leading geneticists as to the possibility of applying modern genetic concepts to the problem of human disease, and especially to the field of psychiatry.

From these general considerations, we shall turn to the question of the dependence of individual nervous and mental diseases upon heredity. We shall make a survey of the important literature bearing upon the subject, paying less attention to the older statistics, in most of which all types of nervous and mental diseases were lumped together indiscriminately, and more to the newer studies which are concentrated upon individual disease entities. Here we shall try to find a middle ground between those who regard every aberration as psychopathic and hereditary, and those who consider all disease to be produced by the environment.

Definition of Sterilization

Sterilization should not be confused with castration or genitalectomy, although in the sterilization laws of some communities castration is still considered as part of the program, while genitalectomy has everywhere disappeared.

The term *sterilization* as used in all modern discussions of eugenics should apply only to the cutting of the vas deferens in the male and the tying off or cutting of the fallopian tubes in the female. We should probably concede that these measures involve no real cruelty since they are carried out under modern surgical conditions and with the standardized surgical technique; furthermore, that these operations do not lower or materially injure sexual power or sexual gratification, nor do they seem to involve a change of personality or a psychic mutilation in most instances. They are the simplest possible permanent devices for excluding the sperm from union with the egg in sexual intercourse.

It should be pointed out that though the avowed purpose of such sterilization invariably starts out by being a eugenic measure, it often ends by becoming a social one. Thus it may be said that individuals who are defective, either by virtue of a genetic constitution or by virtue of some environmental event, may be unable to care for their families, or may be injured in health through the added responsibility.

History of Sterilization

The first sterilization laws were enacted in the United States. The first bill was introduced in the legislature of Michigan in 1897 but failed in passage by a few votes. Two years later, in 1899, Dr. Harry Sharp of the Indiana State Reformatory began systematic sterilization of boys by the then new method of vasectomy. This was done without legal warrant but was the beginning of eugenic sterilization in the United States.

The first sterilization law passed by an American legislature was in Pennsylvania in 1905, but it was vetoed by the governor. The first law was adopted by Indiana in 1907, but in 1909 the governor practically made it impossible of enforcement, and in 1920 it was declared unconstitutional. In 1927, however, it was re-introduced. In 1909 sterilization laws were introduced in California, Washington and Connecticut. Following this, sterilization statutes were adopted in rapid succession by a number of states. Up to the present time the following states have enacted sterilization laws: Alabama, Arizona, California, Connecticut, Delaware, Idaho, Indiana, Iowa, Kansas, Maine, Michigan, Minnesota, Mississippi, Montana, Nebraska, New Hampshire, North Carolina, North Dakota, Oklahoma, Oregon, South Dakota, Utah, Vermont, Virginia, Washington, West Virginia and Wisconsin. Many of these laws were enacted without any definite program. They were frequently changed, revised, vetoed, and amended, and in many instances fell into disuse. Some of them have never really been put into effect, and the number of operations performed is so small as to be negligible. A few hundred each have been done in Wisconsin, Kansas, Nebraska and Minnesota. California has had, in 1935, almost as many sterilizations on record as the rest of the United States put together, this being the only state where the law has been in operation continuously for twenty-one years. Even here the total number of operations is only relatively large: approximately 9,931, as Gosney and Popenoe report.

In the case of only one state, Virginia, has the sterilization law been declared constitutional by the Supreme Court of the United States. The Virginia case is well known as it called forth the celebrated aphorism of Justice Holmes, "Three generations of imbeciles is enough." He further says, "We have seen more than once that the public welfare may call upon the best citizens for their lives. It would be strange if it could not call upon those who already sap the strength of the state for lesser sacrifices, often not felt to be such by those concerned, in order to prevent our being swamped with incompetence."

Outside of the United States, sterilization laws have been enacted in Denmark, Switzerland (Canton of Vaud), Germany, and Canada, and more recently in the state of Vera

Cruz (Mexico), Sweden, Norway, and Finland. The first Canadian law, introduced in 1928, provided for voluntary sterilization of the inmates of state hospitals. In Europe the first sterilization was performed in Switzerland in 1907 but without any legal warrant. The technique used was castration. England has discussed the sterilization law for years, but with true British caution has not yet reached a decision.

The history of the eugenic movement in Germany has been strongly tinged with the belief in Nordic and, more especially, German superiority, but the sterilization program which finally became enacted is a definite attempt to eliminate those diseases which authoritative German psychiatry and eugenics have declared to be hereditary.

II

THE LAWS

THE laws are here briefly analyzed in respect to the following points: first, date of passage; second, to whom applied and whether or not for social, as well as eugenic, purposes; third, whether voluntary or compulsory; and fourth, thoroughness of application to the individuals involved by the wording of the law.

These points are selected for the following reasons: first, to discover whether or not there is any discrimination in the intent of the law. Thus, the limitation of the law to persons in state institutions eliminates those whose cacogenesis is as great but who happen to be cared for at home or in private institutions. Second, the word *voluntary* is frequently a mere subterfuge, in that it is often a condition of discharge from the institution that the patient be sterilized, and consequently the individual involved is in the position of being confined or confinable until he gives his consent for sterilization, which hardly makes the bargain free and equal and nullifies the real meaning of the word voluntary. Furthermore, the term *compulsory,* as will be seen, cannot be taken literally when the number of the sterilized is nowhere near the number of people involved by the act of the legislature. The number sterilized throws light on the handicaps of the authorities in the carrying out of the law and, consequently, gives indirect knowledge of the public sentiment of the community. In general, vasectomy and salpingectomy are the only two operations followed. In some states the law permits asexualization which, however, is rarely enforced.

With the American states we consider the Canadian provinces, Alberta and British Columbia:

1. Alberta. The law was passed on March 21, 1928. It applies to any inmate of a mental hospital or a school for mental defectives when being discharged. The law is non-compulsory. When the patient is not capable of giving the consent, that of the husband, wife, parents, or guardian must be obtained. 205 operations have been performed during the entire period to 1934, 157 females and 48 males. The law is not strictly eugenic, in that heredity does not have to be proved, and in fact only 62% of the female cases and 58.8% of the male cases had a psychopathic heredity. The number of cases indicates that the law is only sparsely enforced.

2. British Columbia. This province has passed a sterilization act, but no report has come as to the working of the law or the number of persons sterilized.

3. Alabama. The law was passed in 1919 and amended in 1923. It applies only to the feebleminded and to the inmates of the Partlow State School for Mental Defectives. The law is compulsory. Social reasons enter into its application. There were 210 operations up to January, 1935, on 124 males and 86 females. Obviously, the law is doing little, since this is about 17 sterilizations a year.

4. Arizona. The law was passed in 1929. It applies to any inmate of a state hospital for the insane who is insane, idiotic, imbecilic, feebleminded, or epileptic, and by the laws of heredity is the probable potential parent of socially inadequate offspring likewise afflicted, and if the welfare of the inmate and society would be promoted by such sterilization. This law is definitely eugenic, and it is compulsory. 20 operations have been performed up to January, 1935, 10 males and 10 females. Obviously, this law is a dead letter.

5. California. Laws were passed on June 25, 1909 and on July 27, 1917. The law provides for compulsory asexualization upon discharge of any inmate of a state hospital for the insane or a state home for the feebleminded if afflicted with mental disease which may have been inherited and which is likely to be transmitted to the descendants; the feebleminded of various grades; those suffering from perversions and marked departures from normal mentality, or from diseases of a syphilitic nature at the discretion of the state commission in lunacy. The law further provides for asexualization of recidivist criminals, if they have been found guilty three times of any crime or crimes, twice for rape or assault with intent to commit rape or seduction, upon the discretion of the resident physician of any state prison, the general superintendent of state hospitals, and the secretary of the state board of health, if the procedure is considered beneficial and conducive to the benefit of the physical, mental, and moral condition of the convict, or any idiot, with the legal consent of his guardian.

While asexualization is permitted, only sterilization is performed. Though the law is compulsory, practically, sterilization in Californian institutions is usually performed with the consent of the patient, husband, wife or next of kin. Although the state has the power to protect itself by compulsion when necessary, the consent of the family is given so readily, in most instances, that it need not be used. It will also be noticed that there is class discrimination in the law, since the patients in private hospitals are exempt from it, as are the patients cared for at home. In other words, the social and financial status also plays a role, the theory being that when an individual becomes an object of public support, he comes under the operation of public measures.

Operations numbering 9,931 have been performed up to January, 1935, 5,147 males and 4,784 females in approximately 26 years, which makes roughly an average of somewhat over 350 cases a year. Although this is the state in which the law is most thoroughly enforced and has become the paradigm of the country, it will be obvious that even here its application is very limited when compared to the extent of the problem.

The Human Betterment Foundation, which is in charge of the propaganda in relationship to sterilization in California and for that matter in this country, is prolific in publications. Thus, one of these publications states that sterilization enables handicapped persons to marry who, without sterilization, would not be able to marry, and that it has been marked by a decrease in sex offenses. One wonders how this has come about, since sterilization does not interfere with the sexual impulse or satisfaction, and it seems a far stretch to believe that sterilization improves sexual morals. In fact, the main objection on the part of many has been that without the fear of pregnancy, sexual offenses would be increased, and it is quite fair to say that the fear of pregnancy is a deterring influence on the conduct of many normal people. It is not probable that feebleminded people commit sex offenses for propagation purposes. It may fairly be stated that much of the propaganda has a journalistic flavor. For example, in Popenoe's and Gosney's book "Sterilization for Human Betterment", the headlines denote that criminality has decreased, but the small print states that, of course, this is not due to sterilization.

6. Connecticut. The law was passed in 1909 and amended in 1919. It applies to persons who, being inmates of a state prison, a state hospital for the insane, or a state training school for the feebleminded, would produce children with an inherited tendency to crime, insanity, feeblemindedness, idiocy or inbecility. The law is compulsory in character. However, it does not authorize a court to order sterilization or to enforce it.

391 operations have been performed up to 1935, 19 males and 372 females, which indicates that the authorities agree

with Kipling that the female of the species is more dangerous than the male. The average number sterilized each year is about 15, which does not indicate that the compulsion is utilized in anything like full power, and so the law is practically non-operative.

7. *Delaware.* The law was passed on April 28, 1932. It applies to the insane, feebleminded, and epileptic for whom procreation is considered inadvisable. Thus, it is eugenic and social. The law is compulsory. 402 operations have been performed up to January, 1935, 184 males and 218 females. The number is too small to be of any significance biologically and indicates that there is no social pressure behind the law.

8. *Idaho.* The law was passed on March 13, 1925 and applies to the feebleminded, insane, epileptic, habitual criminals, moral degenerates, and sexual perverts on the ground that such persons would produce a child or children having an inherited tendency to feeblemindedness, insanity, epilepsy, criminality or degeneracy, or who would probably become a social menace or ward of the state, and who are fundamentally incurable. The law is non-compulsory.

With this magnificent background of application, 14 operations up to January, 1935, have been performed, 4 males and 10 females, so that the law is practically a dead letter.

9. *Indiana.* The law was passed on March 11, 1927 and applies to inmates of state institutions who are insane, idiotic, imbecilic, feebleminded, and epileptic, and who by the laws of heredity are the probable potential parents of socially inadequate offspring likewise afflicted, if they may be sterilized without detriment to the inmate's general health, and if the welfare of the inmate and society would be promoted by such sterilization. The law is compulsory. 353 operations have been performed up to January, 1935, 218 males and 135 females. There has been a definite increase in the past year or two.

We are informed that an attempt is being made to reach the acquired cases of feeblemindedness for purely social and economic reasons. Some judges in the state authorize the sterilization of every feebleminded individual, other judges authorize none, and still other judges are selective, attempting to designate the ones which need sterilization from a hereditary standpoint. The law has been applied almost entirely to the feebleminded.

10. Iowa. The law was passed in April, 1929. It applies to inmates of state institutions for the insane, feebleminded, and epileptic, of the women's reformatory, the penitentiary, and the men's reformatory; in addition, all persons—male or female—living in this state, who are moral degenerates or sexual perverts, who are a menace to society, procreation by whom would produce a child or children having an inherited tendency to feeblemindedness, syphilis, insanity, epilepsy, criminality, or degeneracy, who would probably become a social menace or ward of the state, and who are fundamentally incurable.

It will be seen that this law is, in large measure, social and even takes cognizance of environmental situations, such as syphilis and deals with such vague matters as degeneracy. Out of this scope for the law, 95 operations have been performed up to January, 1935, 57 males and 38 females, which obviously in so populous a state does not indicate a strong popular attitude.

11. Kansas. This is one of the few states in which asexualization is permitted. One law was passed in June, 1913, and the second on May 26, 1917. It is compulsory in operation. It applies to any inmate of a state penitentiary, reformatory, state hospital for the insane, state hospital for epilepsy, state home for the feebleminded, industrial school for girls, if the physical or mental condition would be improved thereby, and if procreation would result in defective or feebleminded children with criminal tendencies.

1,244 operations had been performed up to September,

1934, 584 vasectomies, 422 salpingectomies, 187 castrations, and 51 oophorectomies. By January 1, 1935, the total was 1,362 operations, 839 males and 523 females. The castrations have been done on the feebleminded. (It is difficult to see how castration can improve the general state of the individual operated. It is curious to note, however, that it is this state, which has remained dry since the repeal of the prohibition enactment, which rather sadistically, perhaps, practices asexualization.) Obviously, however, the law is not being thoroughly enforced, since the number so treated has been about 60 a year.

12. Maine. The law was passed July 11, 1925. It applies to any person who is liable to produce further feebleminded offspring or for the therapeutic treatment of certain forms of mental disease. This is on a voluntary basis. Under the compulsory law, any inmate of an institution for the care of the insane and feebleminded, if he would be likely, if released, to produce a child or children who would have the inherited tendency to mental disease or deficiency, must be sterilized.

85 operations have been performed up to January 1, 1935, 7 males and 78 females. We are informed that there is very little opposition to sterilization measures. Most of the operations have been performed under the voluntary law. The laws are administered so as to avoid widespread opposition in principle, and the only opposition encountered is of a religious nature. The law differs from most in that it applies to persons outside of institutions. It will be seen that it is selective in its administration. On the whole, the law is entirely eugenic, but is not thoroughly enforced.

13. Michigan. The law was passed on May 9, 1923. It applies to any mentally defective person, including all feebleminded, insane, epileptic, idiots, imbeciles, moral degenerates and sexual perverts, who would be likely to procreate children with a tendency to mental defectiveness, and if there is no probability that the condition of said defective person would improve, and if it is for the best interest of such person and society that he should be sexually sterilized, because he would be likely, if allowed to mingle in society, to procreate children having an inherited tendency to feeblemindedness, insanity, idiocy, imbecility, epilepsy, or sexual degeneracy, and would be likely to become a social menace or ward of the state, and if there is no probability that the condition of such person would improve to such an extent as to avoid such consequences.

The law is compulsory, but also provides for sterilization with consent. 1,239 operations have been performed up to January, 1935, 307 males and 932 females. In the twelve years of operation the rate has been about 100 a year which, of course, under so inclusive a law in a populous state cannot be said to be highly effective.

14. Minnesota. The law was passed on April 8, 1925. It applies to any person who has been lawfully committed as feebleminded through the guardianship of the state board of control and any person committed as insane to the custody of the superintendent of the state hospital for the insane who has been an inmate of such hospital for at least six consecutive months.

The law is voluntary, but the recommendations are made by the state board of control. 971 operations have been performed up to January, 1935, 113 males and 858 females. We are informed that the board of control never makes a bargain with a family, but also that, practically speaking, the working of the law comes down to this—the higher grade girls and boys in institutions know, as well as do their families, that sterilization is necessary before release becomes easy or possible. Thus, the slogan of the state board of control, indirectly expressed and with many reservations, is—the price of freedom is sterilization. The voluntariness may seriously be questioned, at least from an ethical point of view. Moreover, to some extent, some persons are kept longer in institutions than they might otherwise be, due to the fact that they will not give consent to sterilization. This probably occurs throughout the country.

15. Mississippi. The law was passed on April 26, 1928. It is compulsory, but according to information received is carried out on a voluntary basis, and in case of refusal, operation is not performed. The law comes under the jurisdiction of the Mississippi State Hospital and applies to an inmate or patient who is afflicted with recurrent insanity, idiocy, imbecility, feeblemindedness, or epilepsy of a hereditary nature, and who by the laws of heredity is the probable potential parent of socially inadequate offspring likewise afflicted; and who may be sexually sterilized without detriment to his general health; and whose welfare and that of society will be promoted by such operation for sexual sterilization. Up to January 1, 1935, 163 sterilizations have been performed, 27 males and 136 females.

16. Montana. The law was passed on March 15, 1923. It applies to the feebleminded, insane, epileptic, and hereditary idiots, who are inmates of custodial institutions, and provides for eugenic sterilization, both on a compulsory and a voluntary basis.

A total number of 59 operations on inmates of the school for feebleminded, 25 for the state school for the insane, had been performed up to August, 1934, that is, 84 in all. Since then, the total has reached 85. It will be seen that the statute is not being fully enforced, since there is an average of less than 8 operations per year.

17. Nebraska. A law was passed on July 8, 1915 that the insane and feebleminded should be sterilized before parole or discharge, provided written consent was obtained; in other words, this law was voluntary and applied until 1929. The present law was passed in 1929 and is compulsory for the feebleminded before leaving institutions and non-compulsory for the insane before being discharged or paroled from a state hospital. Up to January, 1935, the total number of operations had reached 276, 112 males and 164 females. The law is being enforced better than in most states but not to a degree of great eugenic importance on any theory.

18. New Hampshire. The first law was passed in 1917 and applied to inmates of a county institution who were insane, feebleminded, or epileptic, on a voluntary basis. The present law was passed in April, 1929, is compulsory, and applies to any inmate of a state or county institution afflicted with hereditary forms of insanity which are recurrent; idiocy, imbecility, feeblemindedness, or epilepsy, and who by the laws of heredity is the probable potential parent of socially inadequate offspring likewise afflicted. The first law was relatively a dead letter. At the state school for feebleminded 11 males and 60 females have been sterilized. The total number up to January, 1935, is 199; 29 males and 170 females. Sterilization in the case of the feebleminded is confined to the higher imbeciles and morons who can go out on their own responsibility and earn their living if without the encumbrance of children.

The authorities are optimistic. They state, "Selective sterilization cuts off definitely hereditary lines. It grants greater social liberty to the individual. It relieves the community of the support of probable defective offspring. . . . While we know little of heredity, like begets like in a general way, as it always did and as it always will, and sterilization is the only bit of preventive medicine we are exercising." Obviously, the female is held to represent the greater potential danger to the community. However, it cannot be stated that the law is sternly enforced, since in 17 years the number sterilized has been small.

19. North Carolina. The first law was passed on February 16, 1929 and declared unconstitutional in February, 1933. Under this law 49 operations were performed, on 13 males and 36 females. The present law was passed in 1933. It is compulsory, and applies to any mentally diseased, feebleminded or epileptic person in and outside of state institutions, if he or she would be likely to procreate a child, or children, who would have a tendency to serious physical, mental, or nervous disease or deficiency. 114 operations have been performed up to January, 1935, on 29 males and 85 females. Public sentiment in this state is said to be favorable to the law.

20. North Dakota. The first law was passed on March 13, 1913, and the present law in 1927. The law is compulsory and applies to the feebleminded, the insane, the epileptic, habitual criminals, moral degenerates, and sexual perverts, who are inmates of state institutions, the state penitentiaries, state hospitals for the insane, state training school, and the state hospitals for the feebleminded, and who are potential to producing offspring who, because of inheritance of inferior or anti-social traits, would probably become a social menace or wards of the state. 150 operations have been performed since 1913, 60 males and 90 females up to January, 1935; at the Grafton State School up to October 1, 1934, 69 females and 5 males have been operated upon; and at the state training school in Mandan about five operations a year are performed at the present time.

Although the law is compulsory, it has been conducted on a voluntary basis, yet with the same compulsion of being a prelude to discharge or parole from an institution. On the whole, the cause of eugenics is not being thoroughly served in the state.

21. Oklahoma. The law was passed on April 22, 1931, is compulsory, and applies to inmates in state institutions for the insane before discharge, who are afflicted with hereditary forms of insanity that are recurrent; idiocy, imbecility, feeblemindedness, or epilepsy. Very few operations have been performed, and only in state institutions for the insane. Up to January, 1935, 8 operations have been performed, 1 male and 7 females. The law is practically a dead letter.

22. Oregon. The law was passed on February 24, 1923 and amended on February 25, 1925 and provides for sterilization, with or without consent. It applies to all persons, male or female, who are feebleminded, insane, epileptic, habitual criminals, moral degenerates or sexual perverts, who are likely to become a menace to society and who would produce a child or children with a tendency to feeblemindedness, epilepsy, insanity, criminality, or perversion, or who would be likely to become a social menace or ward of the state. 957 operations have been performed up to January, 1935, 309 males and 648 females.

Sterilization is not performed without consent of parents, husband, or wife, or nearest of kin, or legal guardian. While the state has the power to protect itself by compulsory operation when necessary, the consent of the family is usually so easy to obtain that court action has not been necessary. "Experience has demonstrated that by preventing procreation of the unfit of this state, this law has been successful in preventing the procreation of many unfit persons."

23. South Dakota. The law was passed on March 8, 1917, and was re-enacted on July 1, 1919. It is compulsory and applies to inmates of state institutions who may be the parents of diseased, feebleminded, idiotic, or imbecilic offspring. Up to January, 1935, 215 operations have been performed, 74 males and 141 females.

24. Utah. The present law was passed in 1929. It applies to inmates of the state hospital, of the state training school, of the state industrial school, or of the state prison, who are afflicted with habitual degenerate sexual criminal tendencies, insanity, idiocy, imbecility, feeblemindedness, or epilepsy. The law is compulsory. Up to January, 1935, 85 operations have been performed, 44 females and 41 males. It will be seen that the law has not been strictly enforced.

25. Vermont. The law was passed in 1931 and is voluntary. It applies to any idiot, imbecile, feebleminded or insane person who would be likely to procreate idiots, imbeciles, feebleminded, or insane persons. 97 operations have been performed up to January, 1935, 65 females and 32 males, of whom 79 were in institutions and 18 outside of institutions.

26. Virginia. The law was passed on March 29, 1924. It is compulsory and applies to any inmate of a state institution who is insane, idiotic, imbecilic, feebleminded, or epileptic, and who by the laws of heredity is the probable potential parent of socially inadequate offspring likewise afflicted. 1,914 operations have been performed up to January, 1935, 755 males and 1,159 females.

27. Washington. The present law was passed on March 8, 1921. It applies to inmates of state institutions who are feebleminded, insane, epileptic, habitual criminals, moral degenerates and sexual perverts, who are persons potential to producing offspring who, because of inheritance of inferior or anti-social traits, would probably become a social menace or wards of the state. The law is voluntary. 30 operations have been performed up to January, 1935, 24 females and 6 males. Very little has been accomplished under this act, due to the failure of the legislature to appropriate funds necessary for carrying on the work.

28. West Virginia. The law was passed in 1929 and is compulsory. It applies to inmates of state institutions who are afflicted with any hereditary form of insanity that is recurrent, idiocy, imbecility, feeblemindedness, or epilepsy, and who by the laws of heredity is the probable potential parent of socially inadequate offspring likewise afflicted. 10 females have been sterilized up to January, 1935. The law has rarely been enforced in this state, because the procedure required to sterilize an individual is too complicated to be carried out.

29. Wisconsin. The law was passed on July 31, 1913. The law is neither outspokenly compulsory nor definitely non-compulsory. It is, however, as to its formulation generally considered compulsory. It applies to inmates of state or county institutions who are criminal, insane, feebleminded, or epileptic, for whom procreation is inadvisable. 645 operations have been performed up to January, 1935, 576 females and 69 males. The state authorities inform us that "The practical application of the law has been too limited. The main province for compulsory human surgical sterilization is in the field of the criminal mentally deficient. It has been applied for the most part to the non-delinquent mentally deficient. Use of the law has been so restrained because the state had no proper place for the detention of mentally deficient criminals prior to sterilization, nor legal provision for their parole under proper supervision subsequent to sterilization."

Summary of American and Canadian laws

It will be seen that in the main these laws, whether on a compulsory or a voluntary basis, are not being enforced, with the exception of a very few states, notably California. The number sterilized is of no great biologic or social significance and fails to fulfill in a large way either social or eugenic aims or needs.

Furthermore, there is no definition of the types of mental disease which are hereditary, and consequently the word "insanity" appears. The German law is far more precise and better drawn up in this respect, since it names schizophrenia and manic-depressive psychosis as sterilizable conditions, and thus has reached clinical precision. It is obvious that the term insanity means nothing from a psychiatric point of view, and since the enforcement of the laws rests upon the opinions of psychiatrists, there should be a conformity to present day psychiatric classification. In the later discussion, it will be clear that very few of the mental diseases can be placed on a hereditary basis and that, consequently, whatever eugenic basis there is for sterilization should be definitely related to present day knowledge or opinion.

Furthermore, the American laws mainly, almost inevitably, concern individuals in state hospitals, and very often it becomes a condition of their discharge that they are sterilized. If the eugenic situation is of importance, there should be no limitation to individuals in state hospitals. If the need of sterilization is financial, then that should be clearly stated. The laws are discriminatory, and while we defer judgment at the present moment as to the need of sterilization, it is simple justice to state that if legislation is necessary, then it should be applied to individuals confined in private institutions and wherever possible to individuals who are not in hospitals at all, but who are mentally sick and whose offspring might inherit their defect.

Foreign Laws

Denmark. The law was passed in June, 1929, and applies to sexual criminals who are considered abnormal and who are in institutions of the prison type. It also applies to mentally abnormal persons in appropriate institutions. The request for sterilization must follow medical advice and receive official sanction by the Minister of Justice who makes certain that the person concerned, or his guardian, clearly understands the nature of the operation which is to be performed.

According to the report of the British Commission, 40 women in institutions for the feebleminded and 14 men in the Detention Institution have been sterilized. The operation in the case of the men is complete bilateral castration. It will be seen that the law has been too limited in application to be of any fundamental value and that there can be no strong public sentiment behind it.

Switzerland (Canton of Vaud). A voluntary law was passed in the Canton of Vaud in January, 1929. It applies to those persons suffering from mental disease, mental infirmity, or drug habituation. The number of operations is very small. According to the last report 29 females have been sterilized, 23 of whom were feebleminded, 3 schizophrenic, 1 manic-depressive, 1 epileptic, and 1 post-encephalitic. A male, described as a feebleminded sex delinquent, was castrated. It is clear that the law is a dead letter, so far as its effectiveness is concerned.

Germany. The most important law which has been passed and put into effect is the German law. This law was enacted on July 14, 1933 and went into effect on January 1, 1934. It is fair to state that it is not a product of the Hitler regime, in that its main tenets were proposed and considered several years before the Nazi regime took possession of Germany. Peter's [1] translation reads:

> Those hereditarily sick may be made unfruitful (sterilized) through surgical intervention when, following the experience of medical science, it may be expected with great probability that their offspring may suffer severe physical or mental inherited damage.
>
> The hereditary sick, in the sense of this law, is a person who suffers from one of the following diseases: inborn feeblemindedness, schizophrenia, circular insanity, hereditary epilepsy, hereditary Huntington's chorea, hereditary blindness, hereditary deafness, severe hereditary physical deformity. Further, those may be made unfruitful who suffer from severe alcoholism.

It will be seen that this law is very precise and, as appears later, conforms closely with the present knowledge of medical eugenics. The law is hedged around with safeguards and official intervention. Provisions are made for trial, appeal, and execution of the law with characteristic German thoroughness. There are Hereditary Health Courts and Hereditary Supreme Courts. There are officials who are set aside to interpret and enforce the law, in a much more deliberate and complete fashion than is the case in the United States or elsewhere. We have no official data as to the number of people sterilized, and very conflicting statements have been

[1] Peter, W. W.: "Germany's Sterilization Program"; Am. J. of Pub. Health, 24, 3:187-191, March, 1934.

made as to the number sterilized and the popular reaction to the measure.

Norway, Sweden, Finland, and the state of Vera Cruz in Mexico have passed sterilization laws, but so recently that the results have not yet appeared in the report. Other countries which have either proposed or drafted sterilization laws, but which have not yet been put into effect include Tasmania and New Zealand.

III

MAIN ARGUMENTS FOR STERILIZATION

In most of the propaganda for sterilization, the following statements appear which we will discuss *in extenso:*

First, insanity, feeblemindedness, epilepsy, pauperism, alcoholism, and certain forms of criminality are on the increase.

TABLE I.

Patients in Hospitals 1880 to 1929 [1]

Mental Patients in State Hospitals at Beginning of Year

Year	Number	Ratio Per 100,000 General Population	Index of Increase for Each Census (1904 equals 100)	
			In Number	In Ratio
1929	272,527	225.9	210.9	143.0
1928	264,511	222.3	204.7	140.7
1927	256,858	219.0	198.8	138.6
1926	246,486	217.3	190.7	137.5
1923	229,664	207.5	177.7	131.3
1922	222,406	204.0	172.1	129.1
1910	159,096	173.0	123.1	109.5
1904	129,222	158.0	100.0	100.0
1890	67,754	107.6	......	......
1880	31,973	63.7	......	......

This table is frequently cited as an index of this increase,

[1] "Mental Patients in State Hospitals 1926 and 1927"; Washington, Government Printing Office, 1930, p. 6; quoted by J. H. Landman in "Human Sterilization"; The Macmillan Co., New York, 1932, p. 7.

which, it will be seen, is not only in actual numbers but in proportion to the total population. The alarm felt by this increase is echoed throughout the writings of all the eugenists. Thus, Kende states there was an increase in insanity, during the ten years of his study, of 24% in Italy, whereas in the United States the increase was 400%.

Such men as Rüdin, and Whitney, stress the fact that insanity is increasing at a terrific rate and imply quite definitely that the biological unfitness is thus threatening to swamp the race. Joseph Mayer quotes this change in the statistics of the cultural countries as alarming. The writings of Laughlin, Baur, Fischer, Lenz, Mjoen and, practically speaking, all the important books echo these statements and stress eugenic measures as the only possible protection society has against further deterioration.

The second statement made is that these defective people propagate at a greater rate than the normal population. Everywhere in the popular literature on the subject the large families of the feebleminded, of the insane, and of the pauper class are stressed, and it is pointed out that the general birth rate, especially for the people of the higher levels, is declining.

A third argument is that these conditions are fundamentally and mainly hereditary, and it is common to speak of insanity, feeblemindedness, epilepsy, pauperism, and criminality, as if these were unitary traits and at the same time were linked together as a psychopathic set of trends.

Fourth, the proponents of eugenics usually stress the environment as, on the whole, of much less importance than the germplasm in the creation of adverse social status, of mental disease, of criminality and of social maladjustment generally. Implicit and often explicit in their philosophy is the point of view that euthenics, or social amelioration, is against natural selection and keeps alive the unfit, so that ameliorative influence is, generally speaking, against the racial welfare.

Alleged Increase of Mental Diseases and Defective Mentality

We may examine certain of the statements made not as implying that sterilization is or is not indicated, but solely from their truth or provability at the present time. First, that these conditions are on the increase. It is really very difficult to prove that mental diseases of any particular type are on the increase. It may be definitely stated, without any fear of contradiction, *that committability and recognition are on the increase,* although certainly not everywhere. That this increase necessarily reflects a biologic change is hardly credible in view of the rapid rise in the commitment rate in certain places and the general lag in others. Thus, in the southern part of the United States, the commitment rate is nowhere near as high as in the northern part. "For example, in New England, according to the latest statistics, the rate in the mental hospitals per 100,000 population was more than 375; in the South it was less than 150. The states with the highest rates, Massachusetts and New York, had 27 and 46 hospitals respectively; those with the lowest rates, New Mexico, Alabama and Arkansas, had only one or two hospitals each. The accessibility of a hospital will affect the admission rate. For example, a family would readily commit one of its members to a hospital located within a few miles from home, but would hesitate to send him to one more than 100 miles away." [1] These figures and Table I are entirely misleading. They apply not to the admission rates, but to the accumulation rate. Whenever a new hospital is built and as the death rate in the hospital diminishes, there is an accumulation of patients. As the admission figures later show, this is an entirely different matter from the "new patient rate" which more nearly measures the biology of mental disease.

Moreover, in the states where hospital commitments are

[1] Statistical Bulletin, Metropolitan Life Insurance Company, V. 16, no. 2, February, 1935, pp. 6-8.

high, facilities are good, the hospitals are adequate, and the care of the patient is, on the whole, excellent; whereas, in the states where hospitals are few and the commitment rate low, the hospitals are inadequate, poorly equipped, poorly manned, and it would be quite natural for people to hesitate to send their patients there.

Furthermore, there is an interesting correlation between the general care taken of the population and the commitment rate. In Massachusetts and New York, there are far more schools and far more hospitalization facilities for the sick of all kinds than in the states where the commitment rate is low. Moreover, the rate of increase is too rapid to be biologic.

The rate is decidedly greater for urban than for rural districts, which has been interpreted to mean that the city has always been more fertile soil for the seeds of mental disorders than the rural districts, and that the movement of the population into the cities probably results, among other things, in increased incidence of mental disease.

Thus, Pollock and Furbush state, for example, that 71.4% of the commitments in the United States come from urban districts, and 27.1% from rural environments.[1] This may be interpreted in two ways. Generally speaking, the urban districts have better hospitals, more facilities for the detection of the mentally sick, and furthermore, much more interest in mental diseases. A deteriorating schizophrenic or a moron might well adjust himself to farm life, whereas he might be seriously maladjusted in the big city. Urbanization may not mean that more mental disease arises in the urban districts, but merely that it becomes socially more discernible, and the affected individuals become more maladjusted in the cities than in the rural districts.

[1] This is very similar to the statistics of the Massachusetts hospitals where the urban rate is 79 per 100,000 and the rural rate is 25 per 100,000, with the interesting and disturbing fact demonstrated that it is in the villages and the large cities that the higher rates obtain, while it is the smaller cities which furnish the least number of patients per 100,000.

There is a curious contradiction in the statements made about the ill effects of urban and cultural life and the fact that the families which have become classic in the eugenic literature as examples of cacogenics come from rural or semi-rural districts. When one goes into isolated communities, one finds groups of strikingly low intelligence.

To reach a conclusion as to the actual biology of the situation, that is, whether or not there is more mental disease independent of hospital facilities, is a difficult but not insoluble matter. We have selected two states of the union which offer, on the whole, the best testing ground for statistics on the situation. Both in Massachusetts and New York, the hospitals are plentiful; they are not far away from the individuals who need them, and the general social interest has not changed much in the last fifteen or twenty-five years. There are many well-trained men working in each of these communities. Interest in mental hygiene is at its height, and the social conditions upon the whole have been fairly stable so far as hospitals are concerned for almost a generation. This study has been made for the committee by Drs. Henry B. Elkind and Maurice Taylor, the one a psychiatrist with statistical training, and the other a sociologist and statistician.

Tables II and III and Charts I and II, which follow, represent figures and graphs which involve an age correction of the statistics. It is obvious that since there is little mental disease, excluding feeblemindedness and epilepsy, below the age of 15, the population younger than this should not be included in the statistics, especially in view of the fact, which is now well established, that the average age of the population is increasing. Moreover, in order to obtain the correct admission rate for the various mental diseases, their age of incidence must be taken into account. There is little general paresis before the age of 35. There is almost no commitment for psychoses with cerebral arterial disease and for senile psychoses before the age of 55. Therefore, these figures are corrected as follows: *all psychoses* 15 years and over; *general paresis* 35 years and over; *senile psychoses* 55 years and over; *senile psychoses with cerebral arterial disease* 55 years and over; *manic-depressive* and *dementia praecox* separately and jointly 15 years and over. These statistical adjustments are necessary to obtain a true assessment of increase or decrease in admission rate.

We have considered the admissions under the following diagnostic headings: first, manic-depressive psychosis and dementia praecox. These two diseases constitute the endogenous psychoses, so-called, for which at present there is no external or environmental cause established. Moreover, because of the frequently encountered difficulty in the differential diagnosis between these two psychoses and the consequent great liability to error, we have also considered the admission rate of these two psychoses as a unit. It is in these two diseases in which heredity appears to play a great role. Our second group is that of the alcoholic psychoses; a third is general paresis; a fourth is cerebral arteriosclerotic and senile dementias. We have also considered these latter two as a unit, first, because of the age of incidence; second, because the error of diagnosis during life is too great to permit a separation which has any real value.

The tables and charts show that the rise of the population is about paralleled by the rise of admissions of cases of manic-depressive psychosis in the State of Massachusetts. It is at least safe to say that there is no increase in the admissions of this disease. Of New York the same can be stated, although in the last few years there has been a slight rise in the admission rate which, however, does not reach the level of 1927 and 1928.

Dementia praecox shows, in the case of Massachusetts, a decrease in the admission rate; in the case of New York a slight rise, whereas for the previous years the rate is fairly constant, although with some ups and downs. Since the last three years are the depression years, this more likely

FIRST ADMISSIONS (COURT COMMITMENTS ONLY) TO MASSACHUSETTS STATE HOSPITALS AND McLEAN HOSPITAL: RATES PER 100,000 POPULATION (ADJUSTED FOR AGE - SEE TABLE II) FOR THE YEARS 1920-1933 INCLUSIVE -

- CHART I -

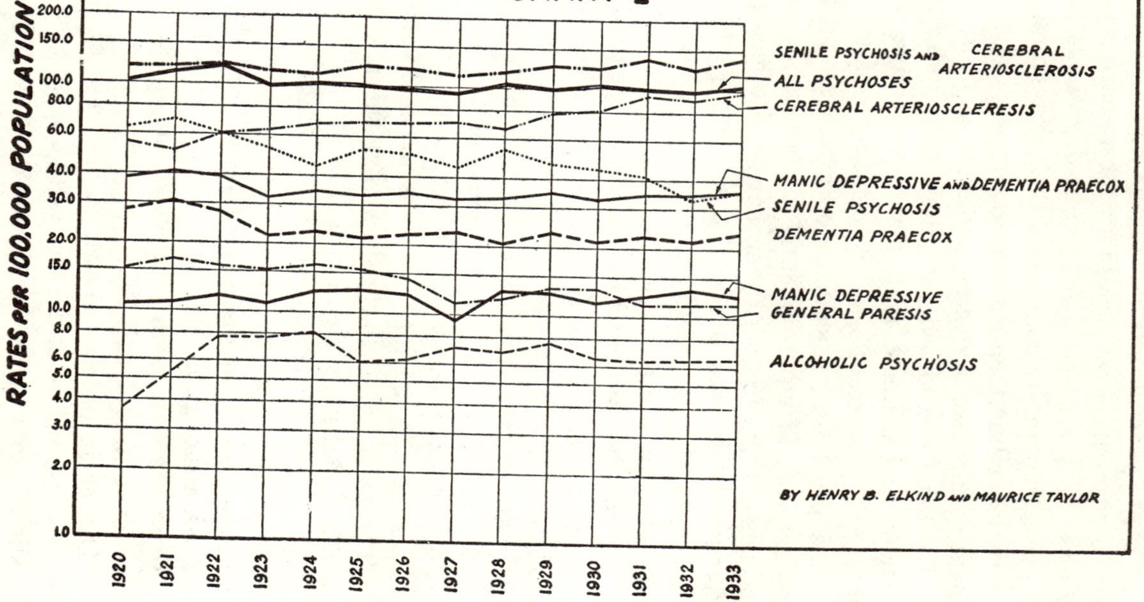

TABLE II.

MASSACHUSETTS

First Admissions (Court commitments only) to Massachusetts State Hospitals and McLean Hospital
Rates per 100,000 Population (adjusted for age) for the years 1920–1933 inclusive.

Rates per 100,000 Population

Year	Population 15 years+				Population 35 years+	Population 55 years+			Population 15 years+
	Alcoholic Psychoses	Dementia Praecox	Manic-depressive	D.P. and M.D.	General Paresis	Senile Psychosis	Cerebral Arterio-sclerosis	S.P. and C.A.	All Psychoses
1920	3.7	27.5	10.6	38.1	15.1	64.0	55.2	119.2	102.0
1921	5.3	30.7	10.8	41.5	16.7	69.0	50.7	119.7	111.0
1922	7.6	27.4	11.7	39.1	15.7	61.0	60.7	121.7	118.0
1923	7.7	21.5	10.9	32.4	15.2	52.0	62.6	114.6	98.0
1924	8.1	22.5	12.4	34.9	16.1	44.0	67.7	111.7	101.0
1925	6.0	21.1	12.6	33.7	15.4	52.0	68.5	120.5	100.0
1926	6.3	22.2	12.1	34.3	14.1	50.0	69.5	119.5	97.0
1927	7.1	23.0	9.4	32.4	11.3	44.0	69.8	113.8	94.0
1928	6.9	20.5	12.7	33.2	11.8	53.0	66.6	118.6	102.0
1929	7.6	23.0	12.6	35.6	13.1	46.0	79.5	125.5	99.0
1930	6.6	21.0	11.4	32.5	13.1	44.0	80.6	124.6	102.0
1931	6.3	22.8	12.3	35.1	11.3	41.0	94.1	135.1	100.0
1932	6.4	21.5	13.2	34.7	11.4	32.5	90.7	123.0	98.5
1933	6.5	23.6	12.4	36.0	11.4	36.0	97.9	133.9	102.0

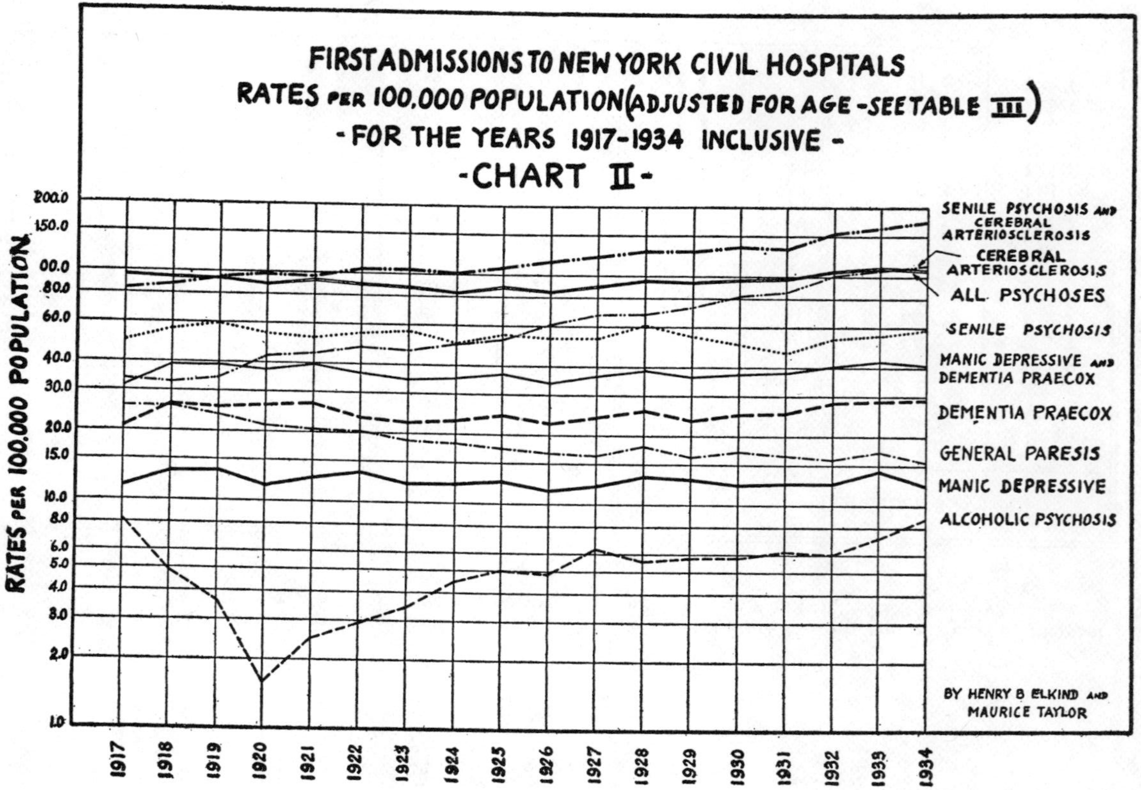
FIRST ADMISSIONS TO NEW YORK CIVIL HOSPITALS
RATES PER 100,000 POPULATION (ADJUSTED FOR AGE - SEE TABLE III)
- FOR THE YEARS 1917-1934 INCLUSIVE -
- CHART II -
RATES PER 100,000 POPULATION
200.0
150.0
00.0
80.0
60.0
40.0
30.0
20.0
15.0
10.0
8.0
6.0
5.0
4.0
3.0
2.0
1.0
1917
1918
1919
1920
1921
1922
1923
1924
1925
1926
1927
1928
1929
1930
1931
1932
1933
1934
SENILE PSYCHOSIS AND CEREBRAL ARTERIOSCLEROSIS
CEREBRAL ARTERIOSCLEROSIS
ALL PSYCHOSES
SENILE PSYCHOSIS
MANIC DEPRESSIVE AND DEMENTIA PRAECOX
DEMENTIA PRAECOX
GENERAL PARESIS
MANIC DEPRESSIVE
ALCOHOLIC PSYCHOSIS
BY HENRY B ELKIND AND MAURICE TAYLOR

TABLE III.

NEW YORK

First Admissions to New York Civil Hospitals
Rates per 100,000 Population (adjusted for age), for the years 1917–1934 inclusive.

Rates per 100,000 Population

Year	Population 15 years+				Population 35 years+	Population 55 years+			Population 15 years+
	Alcoholic Psychoses	Dementia Praecox	Manic-depressive	D.P. and M.D.	General Paresis	Senile Psychosis	Psychosis c Cerebral Arterio-sclerosis	S.P. and C.A.	All Psychoses
1917	8.2	20.3	11.5	31.8	25.4	49.6	33.4	83.0	94.9
1918	4.8	25.7	13.3	39.0	25.6	55.7	33.1	87.8	92.7
1919	3.6	25.2	13.5	38.7	23.6	58.8	33.5	92.3	91.6
1920	1.6	25.6	11.7	37.3	21.1	53.8	42.7	96.5	87.6
1921	2.5	26.6	12.8	39.4	20.5	51.8	44.0	95.8	90.2
1922	2.9	23.2	13.4	36.6	20.1	54.8	47.2	102.0	88.9
1923	3.4	22.4	12.0	34.4	18.7	56.0	46.0	102.0	85.4
1924	4.5	23.1	12.1	35.2	18.2	50.0	50.0	100.0	83.8
1925	5.0	24.1	12.4	36.6	17.4	54.7	53.3	107.0	87.8
1926	4.9	22.5	11.4	33.9	16.9	53.0	61.0	114.0	84.2
1927	6.3	24.2	12.0	36.2	16.5	53.0	67.0	120.0	89.5
1928	5.6	25.7	13.2	38.9	18.0	60.2	68.0	128.0	95.2
1929	5.8	23.4	13.0	36.4	16.3	54.7	73.3	128.0	92.5
1930	5.8	25.0	12.2	37.2	17.1	50.3	81.7	132.0	95.8
1931	6.2	25.3	12.5	37.8	16.6	46.6	85.4	131.0	96.3
1932	6.0	28.1	12.5	40.6	16.0	53.5	101.5	155.0	106.0
1933	7.1	28.5	14.1	42.6	17.2	55.8	108.2	164.0	110.0
1934	8.7	29.0	12.2	41.2	15.4	58.7	113.0	171.7	111.0

represents a social than a biological phenomenon. When the two psychoses, manic-depressive and dementia praecox, are considered together, Massachusetts shows definitely a drop with a flattening of the curve of admissions during the great part of the period considered. In New York there was some increase in the admission rate during the past two years, although it has hardly exceeded the rate reached in 1918, 1919, and 1920.

The case of the alcoholic psychoses is extremely interesting from a social point of view. There was a steady drop in both states from 1917 to 1920. With the passage of the prohibition enactment there was a sharp drop to a very low level, then a steep recovery in the case of Massachusetts until 1922; from then on a rather flat curve indicating a stationary commitment rate. The curve in the case of the New York admissions shows this difference—that from 1920 on, the rise has continued and that at the present time the admission rate practically parallels the rate of increase of the population.

The figures for general paresis, as indicated by the charts, show the following: in Massachusetts there has been a consistent drop in the admission rate for general paresis from 1917 to 1933. In New York state the admission rate has fallen off definitely as compared with the general population.

Throughout the Western world, it has been noted that there has been a marked increase in the number of senile and cerebral arteriosclerotic psychoses. This is by far the most important factor in the increased admission rate. Usually, charts made to represent this increase are plotted against the general population, but this is obviously an error when one takes into account the fact that the number of old people in the community has definitely increased in the past generation; that as the situation has been phrased—the population is getting older. The declining birth rate plus the greater longevity has altered the complexion, so far as age groups are concerned, of Western civilization. We repeat, therefore, that we have plotted our curves against the population of the age of 55 and over rather than of the total population. In Massachusetts the increase of cases of senile dementia and arteriosclerotics as plotted against the population of 55 and over is, on the whole, not significant, since it coincides with depression years. In New York there is a very definite and significant rise of admissions from the year 1924 on. This rise in senile dementia and arteriosclerotic commitments has some plausible social explanations. In the first place, there is the increasing longevity of the population. This is probably the most important factor. Second, as populations grow more urban, it becomes more difficult to care for the elderly who are mentally sick at home. Third, as the hospitals for the mentally sick more nearly approach the complexion of a general hospital, where the senile dementia and arteriosclerotic patient can be cared for in wards which resemble those of any hospital, there is a greater tendency on the part of relatives to commit. They do not feel as if they have abandoned their old people to the lunatic asylum.

We emphasize that we have selected the statistics of Massachusetts as a critical test for the actual increase of mental diseases because Massachusetts has the largest number of beds per 100,000 of its population, more physicians for each patient, a well established and smoothly working state machinery, excellent hospitals, and what is probably just as important, the hospitals are not widely separated from the community which they serve. It is probable that an hour's journey covers the travel necessary from the home of the patient to the hospital. Furthermore, these conditions have operated over a period of time sufficiently long to establish a set of stable circumstances. The conditions in New York closely approach those of Massachusetts, but the building program of New York has lagged behind that of Massachusetts.

We now turn to a comprehensive paper by Ellen Winston, entitled "The Assumed Increase of Mental Disease," whose statistics for the admission rates of many countries are corrected for the age 15 years and over. It will be seen from the tables that the rates of Australia and New Zealand, which were high in 1911, have shown a distinct decline; that in England and Wales, there has certainly been no increase although the curve fluctuates remarkably. The number of first admissions in Scotland has remained, on the whole, the same although with wide fluctuations from year to year. This is also true (although we do not here reproduce the charts) of Norway and the Scandinavian countries. The only cultural country from which good statistics are obtainable and in which there is a marked increase in the admission rate is in Germany, where the rate has gone up from 25 per 100,000 in 1923 to nearly 36 in 1929. *Thus, except for Germany, the same type of curve and the same general peculiarities of admission rates obtain in the European countries as in Massachusetts and New York.* There is an enormous difference between the rates of admission in the various countries, which difference relates undoubtedly more to social and hospital circumstances than to true biology. It is not probable that there is enough biological difference between the people of Australia and New Zealand with their rates ranging from 80–100 per 100,000 and the people of Norway with an average rate of admission around 50, to account for these admission rate differences. The fact that there is a marked increase in the rate of admissions in Germany probably indicates that there is a recently sharpened attention to mental disease in Germany and a growing social concern with the problem. No one, we believe, would seriously contend that Australia has four times as much biological tendency to mental disease as Germany.

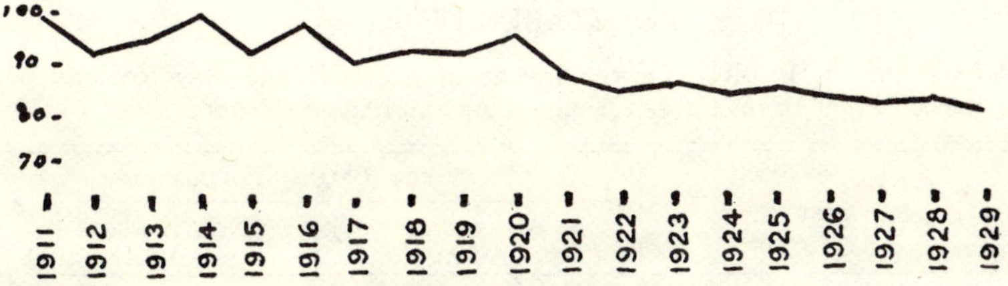

Ratio per 100,000

Fig. 1. Number of admissions to hospitals for the insane in Australia for 100,000 population 15 years of age and over, 1911–29. From E. Winston.

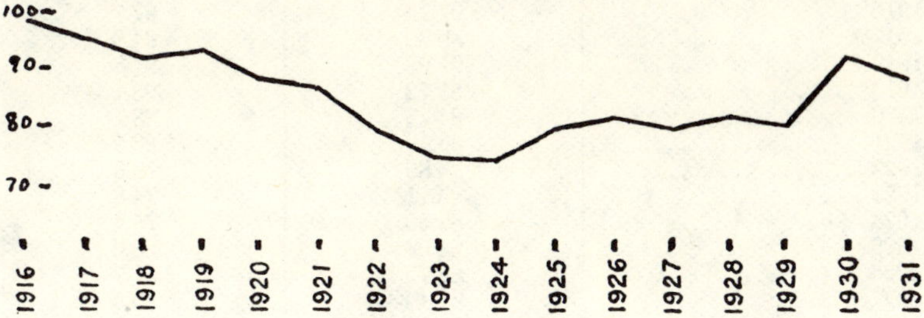

Ratio per 100,000

Fig. 2. Number of first admissions to hospitals for the insane in New Zealand per 100,000 population 15 years of age and over, 1916–31. From E. Winston.

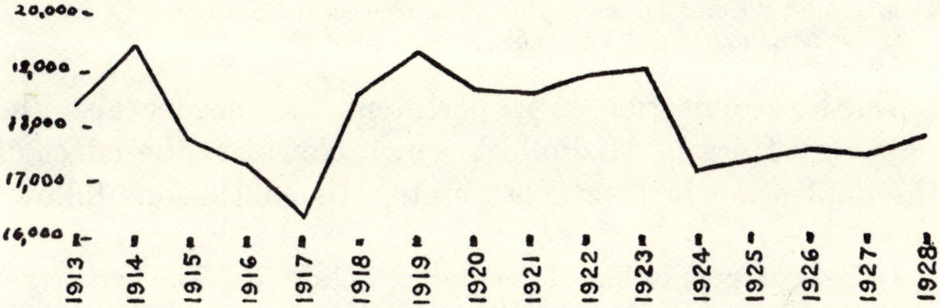

Fig. 3. Number of first admissions to hospitals for the insane in England and Wales, 1913–28. From E. Winston.

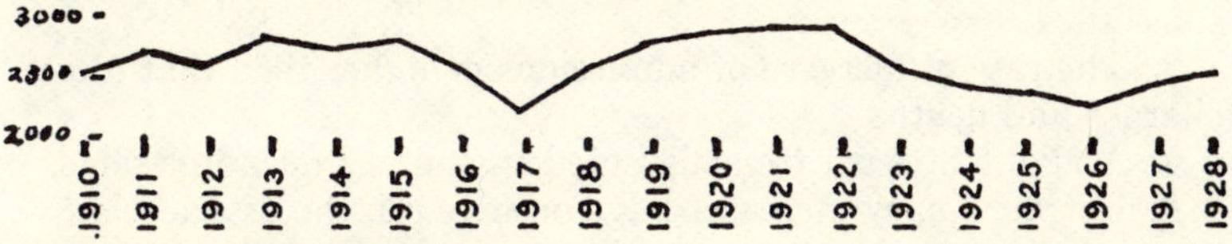

Fig. 4. Number of first admissions to hospitals for the insane in Scotland, 1910–28. From E. Winston.

TABLE IV.

Admissions to Hospitals for the Insane in Australia and New Zealand per 100,000 Population, Fifteen Years of Age and Over (From E. Winston).

Year	Rate per 100,000 Population	
	Australia * (Total Admissions)	New Zealand † (First Admissions)
1911	98.49	....
1912	91.99	....
1913	94.28	....
1914	98.27	....
1915	91.82	....
1916	97.25	97.7
1917	89.72	94.9
1918	91.95	91.8
1919	91.72	93.1
1920	94.73	88.1
1921	86.49	86.8
1922	83.86	79.6
1923	85.11	74.8
1924	82.90	75.4
1925	84.09	80.0
1926	82.72	81.7
1927	81.40	80.5
1928	81.74	82.2
1929	79.24	81.4
1930	.....	92.6
1931	.....	89.0

* Official Yearbook of the Commonwealth of Australia and "Australian Demography," Commonwealth Bureau of Census and Statistics.
† New Zealand, Official Yearbook.

In this connection it is pertinent to consider also the paper by Horatio M. Pollock which considers the effect of the depression in New York state. His conclusions follow:

1. Patient population of mental hospitals in New York state increased more rapidly from 1929 to 1934 than from 1924 to 1929. The increase was greatest in 1933.
2. The trend in the rate of first admissions has been rising since 1924.
3. The rate of increase of admissions is higher than that of discharges and deaths.
4. A slight upward trend is noted in senile first admissions.
5. Extraordinary increases have occurred in the arteriosclerotic group during the past 10 years. The most marked change was in 1932.

6. No change in trend is found in the paretic group.

7. A slowly rising trend is noted in the alcoholic group. The group is more affected by liquor legislation than by economic conditions.

8. The trend in the manic-depressive is slightly upward. A marked increase occurred in this group in 1933.

9. A significant increase in the rate of dementia praecox first admissions has occurred since 1927. The rate was exceptionally high in 1932 and 1933. Such rate may reflect cumulative effects of the depression.

10. The economic crisis does not seem to be the dominant factor in the increase of first admissions in any one diagnostic group; it is, however, a precipitating factor of importance in all groups.

There are several criticisms to be made of the above paper. In the first place, there has been no correction for age incidence in the tables. In the second place, the statement occurs in the text that ever since 1927 a distinct rise in the dementia praecox group has been noted, the most significant change occurring in 1932. The highest rate of first admissions of that year was exceeded by that of 1933. However, when one takes the curve as a whole and corrects it for age, the rate has been up and down with slight variations since 1918.

We quote in this relationship the opinion of a statistical group:

"The decreasing birth rate and the prolongation of life have brought about a greater percentage of older people in the population. The majority of mental cases occurs at the older ages, and the aging of the population would in itself tend to increase the number of mental patients, without really implying any greater tendency for people to become so afflicted." [1]

A factor of importance also is that in a more isolated and primitive community a disorderly, untidy old person can be readily cared for, whereas he becomes quite disorganizing in his tenement or apartment house district and especially where the people of the house go out to work.

[1] Statistical Bulletin of the Metropolitan Life Insurance Company, v. 16, no. 2, February, 1935, p. 7.

An increasing sensitiveness to the care and burden of such old persons goes with the increasing sensitiveness to dirt and disorder which is characteristic of progress. The greater care given these patients in a modern hospital makes it emotionally possible for a family to commit the case of senile dementia or arteriosclerotic deterioration, whereas in a hospital with less care, where the patient would be neglected, the commitment rate of these elderly and aged persons would be low.

The Propagation Rate of the Mentally Diseased and Defectives and Allied Matters

Evidently the propagation rate can be definitely studied from the standpoint of the birth rate, the marriage rate, and the selective death rate of the mentally sick and defective. Is there any statistical proof for such statements as commonly appear, namely, that the birth rate of the defectives is high; that they tend biologically to increase because their relative fertility and survival is greater than that of the normal? If the birth rate, marriage rate and death rate are studied by isolated family reports, then alarm may be felt, but if the statistics as a whole are considered, a curious, not easily explainable, *complete contradiction* to the statements usually made in the eugenic literature appears.

Alarming statements that need to be considered are, for example, those made by Lenz who states that the abnormal propagate twice as rapidly as the normal population, but since Lenz states definitely that the ugly are abnormal as compared to the handsome, and since he seems to consider the Nordic type as handsome, his statement may be taken with some degree of skepticism, especially by those who do not happen to be handsome or Nordic.

O'Gorman also states that the fertility of the abnormal is two to six times as great as the normal, and somewhat more conservatively Dirksen writes that the abnormal have on the average 8.8 to 4 children, while the normals have only 5 to 2. He lumps together the feebleminded, insane, and criminal as abnormal under the heading of asocial, and his work does not seem to be specific or detailed.

When we come down to the actual studies that have been made on the marriage rates, the birth rates, and the death rates of known groups of the insane and feebleminded, we find quite a different complexion to the situation, one not so alarming and, in fact, quite reassuring. Even Popenoe, who is the leading practical worker in the field of eugenical sterilization in the United States, in discussing the marriage rates states:

1. The marriage rate of the psychotic of both sexes is markedly below that of the general population of all ages.

2. While the male psychotics marry freely (though in diminished proportion) at all ages, the female marriage rate remains almost constant after the age of thirty.

3. Since three-fourths of all first admissions are aged thirty or over, it appears that a woman, who is single on admission to a hospital for mental diseases is, even if promptly discharged, likely to remain single during the rest of her life.

4. A far-reaching program of sterilization must, therefore, find some way of dealing with these women in the pre-psychotic stage.

5. There is some indication that in women, the lower marriage rate is partly due to deliberate abstention from marriage, and not merely to failure to attract a mate.

6. Wide differences exist in the marriage rates of men with various types of psychosis.

7. The same variation is found in women, but one-third less than in men.

8. The marriage rate of sterilized patients with dementia praecox is lower than that of the manic-depressives at all ages. The two curves do not show any other striking disparity.

9. In a small group of males with dementia praecox, the percentage having more or less normal heterosexual libido is much larger than has been reported in previous studies.

Myerson asks the following question:

Do the psychoses interfere with the marriage rate, or rather does the condition underlying a psychosis—alcoholism, syphilis, psychopathic constitution—interfere with marriage?

Summarizing the results, we find first, that the males in the alcoholic, paretic, and dementia praecox groups marry less than do the females. In the seniles, though the percentage of married men is greater, the totals of those who have entered conjugal relations at one time or other are about equal. Looking somewhat closer, it is found that in paresis there is only a slight difference in favor of the female. In alcoholics there is a very decided difference in favor of the female, and in dementia praecox this difference is still further increased. Thus, if these groups may be held to constitute a menace by virtue of their ability to transmit the psychotic taint to another generation, the female of the species, to use a well-known phrase, is more dangerous than the male.

It will be seen that in the four diseases the females marry in about the same ratio, except in the case of dementia praecox where the falling off is considerable. In the males, there is much more decided irregularity in marriage ratios, whereas the seniles and the general paretics marry but slightly less than do the same age groups in the total population, while the male dementia praecox has an exceedingly low marriage rate. *That is, whatever is back of dementia praecox operates against self-perpetuation.* Something of the same internal mechanism is seen in the case of alcoholic psychoses. This mechanism operates very little, if at all, in the case of paresis and the senile psychoses. One might conclude that if there is an inborn defect in these diseases it is by far greatest in dementia praecox, is next in alcoholic insanity, and least of all in syphilis and the senile psychoses. And in a general way this will be found to correspond with the belief of the average psychiatrist. For most of us, despite some writers, paresis is held to be wholly an exogenous disease caused by the spirochaeta pallida working on a relatively intact organism. If Koller's and Diem's figures form any criterion, senile psychoses represent conditions that are largely exogenous in their origin. Alcoholic insanity in most clinics is held to be the result of exogenous and endogenous factors, while dementia praecox is believed to be largely of endogenous origin.

Pollock and Furbush, studying the statistics of the United States find that 60.9% of the schizophrenics, 59.3% of the epileptic psychotics, 76.4% of the mentally deficient groups are unmarried. Whatever the illegitimacy rates may be, it may be safely stated that the mental disease groups do not figure disproportionately in them, although this may not be true of the feebleminded. However, illegitimacy as a source of the population is trifling as compared with marriage, and we may safely state that insofar as the opportunity to propagate the race is concerned, those groups which are definitely known to be feebleminded and insane are, in large part, debarred by the fact that they do not tend to marry.

When we come to the question of the size of families, the alarming statements made in the literature do not seem borne out by actual studies. It is true that if one takes isolated examples, one finds many large families in the low grade groups. As has been stated elsewhere low cultural level and mental disease cannot be held to be synonymous, nor is high cultural status, in the sense of wealth and prosperity, coincident with mental hygiene.

Dahlberg found in a large group of women who had been in the insane asylum of Upsala that their fertility was only little more than half of the fertility of normal women from an average population.

Rüdin found that in his group of siblings who had one schizophrenic parent, the number was 29% less per family than in the group in which both parents were phenotypically healthy. There was a 29% decrease in the birth rate if one of the parents was schizophrenic.

Even Popenoe's own figures indicate that in the case of those who are committed to institutions the mean size of families is:

1. For married men 1.64 living children, married women 2.03; all men 0.61, all women 1.85.

2. A married unsterilized insane woman will, on the average, produce a living child every 15 years.

3. The fecundity of the unsterilized insane studied as controls is lower than the above figures. It appears that only one-sixth of

the married female controls will produce enough children to increase the size of their group.

4. In general, no large group of institutional insane in California will produce enough children wholly to reproduce itself, even if it were not sterilized, the completed family being only two or three children. (Higher figures have been reported elsewhere.)

5. Most of the insane are born of parents who are not themselves insane. The fecundity of these parents appears from other studies to be a little greater than that of insane parents. Any extensive program of eugenic sterilization should find a way to reach these parents, at least through making voluntary sterilization possible, if it is to achieve maximum results.

6. There are no significant differences between the sizes of families of sterilized women with the different types of psychoses.

7. Among sterilized married women, the Protestants were found to have about one-third of a living child more than the Roman Catholics. There was no demonstrated difference among the men.

8. Women who had no near relatives insane had each about one-third of a living child more than those who had a family history of mental disease. There was no demonstrated difference among the men.

9. Among insane women in general (married controls of this study), about one-third are childless. Reasons are given for believing that this represents in part a physiological sterility, with which menstrual disturbances are associated.

10. Insane women who had the largest number of living children also tended to have the largest number of dead children.

We quote the above *in extenso* because it represents the statistics gathered by one who is emphatic about the need for sterilization, yet whose own figures insofar as those actually insane are concerned show very definitely that those who are mentally sick to the point of commitment do not anywhere near tend to reproduce themselves.

There is a classical experiment carried on inadvertently and unwillingly by Walter E. Fernald who cites his results in an excellent paper in relation to the marriage rate and the fecundity of the feebleminded on the discharged Waverley patients. There were discharged from his institution in twenty-five years (1890 to 1914) 1,537 patients, of whom 646, 470 males and 176 females, were in the community and could be studied. These 1,537 people were, in the majority of cases, dismissed under protest, as it is the policy of the school to insist on permanent segregation.

Of the 646 people 82 had died, and 101 were readmitted to the school. Of the 176 females, 27 had married and there were as issue 50 children, and of these 17 had died leaving 33 children, which hardly looks like the "remarkable fertility of the feebleminded." Seven of the married women had no children. Nearly all of the married women had married men above their own social status and that of their own parents, that is, these feebleminded women had advanced socially. Of the 27 married women 11 had done well, and 16 had behaved badly, being sexually promiscuous, etc. Of the 176 females there were 11 unmarried mothers, with 13 illegitimate children. None of these had been supervised and most were returned to the hospital. "Apparently the discharged female patients have not contributed largely to the sex and venereal problem, but this is undoubtedly due to the school training and the supervision of relatives. In fact, of the 90 discharged females now in the community 52 are apparently giving no trouble, though needing supervision." Of the 470 males, 13 had married and have 12 children. No comment necessary. "There was a surprisingly small amount of criminality, sex offense, and especially of illegitimacy."

In a similar study Woodall traces the fate of 385 children of 192 feebleminded mothers who had been patients at the Walter E. Fernald School for the Feebleminded. His results are summarized as follows:

1. Out of 385 children of 192 mothers who were patients of the Walter E. Fernald State School, 128 died and most of these died in infancy.

2. Examinations were obtained on 119 children. The mental level of these children ranged from imbecile to superior men-

tality. 16% were of average or superior mentality. 44% were mentally defective. The average mental level of the children was superior to that of the mothers.

3. The general physique of the children exceeded that of the mothers and the children correlated well with their individual mothers in this respect.

4. There was a high positive correlation between the I.Q.'s of mothers and children. This correlation was most marked in those mothers who appeared to be of the hereditary defective type.

Moreover, Popenoe, as well as Brugger, shows that the feebleminded tend, on the whole, to come from the normal middle groups of the population:

The parents of the sterilized patients are distributed (within certain limits) about the same as the whole adult male population of the State of California. Apparently the greatest number of institutional feebleminded are the children of skilled laborers, not of paupers or of the casual labor class. The same is true of the retarded school children of Munich. . . . While the parentage of the sterilized patients is fairly representative of California as a whole, the small intellectual stratum which produces most of the bright children in the public schools, furnishes much less than its quota of mental deficiency.

And continuing in this analysis, Popenoe concludes,

Since the type of feeblemindedness requiring institutional care is found to be so widely distributed throughout the whole population, this study supports the view that the selection of any socio-economic level for sterilization is not an adequate or a scientific procedure. Sterilization must be applied on the merits of each individual case.

While his conclusion is certainly correct insofar as the selection of the persons to be sterilized is concerned, it is equally true that the production of these feebleminded is not by the feebleminded groups; that these individuals represent more or less unknown products of apparently normal people; that there is nothing to show any great prolificity either in their ancestors or in themselves; and, in fact, all the data are against this view. It is only when one considers as representative of the feebleminded such families as the Nams, the Kallikaks, the Jukes, the Hill-Folk, the Zero family, and like social monstrosities that one reaches the opinion that there is a menace in the prolificity of the feebleminded.

Myerson and Elkind, in studying the size of the families from which the feebleminded in institutions come, state that it is only in the case of those relatively few individuals in whom both parents are feebleminded that the family tends to be larger than that of the average population, and that there is nothing to show that the families from which the majority of the feebleminded come are any larger than that of the average population. It is probable that the larger size of the families in these institutional cases is more related to the cultural status of the group than to biologic status, since they represent in large measure the poorer and more recently Americanized groups in which the birth rate on the whole tends to be rather higher than that of the total population.

In the celebrated report of the British Commission, the following blunt statement occurs:

> There is a widespread belief that one of the characteristics common to defectives is abnormal fertility. This is not borne out either by the inquiry or by such other statistics we have been able to collect bearing upon the size of the families of known defectives. . . . It would be easy, though it would serve no useful purpose, to cite cases of excessive fertility; but we are convinced that these cases are exceptional and prove nothing except the terrible results of leaving at large a type of defective wholly unfitted for community life. Except for a relatively small number of isolated instances, we find that there is no evidence of excessive fertility, and indeed it would be easy to set off against these exceptional cases a much larger number of cases in which the fertility rate was low. The supposed abnormal fertility of defectives is, in our view, largely mythical. . . .

That the stability of the marriages of the psychotic or those who become psychotic is very much less than the marriages of the general population is confirmed by Popenoe, who states:

In American institutions in 1922, there were 71 married persons per 100,000 married persons in the whole population, but 320 divorcees per 100,000 of that status outside. In other words, actual mental disease occurs at least four or five times as often among divorcees as among married persons. This is partly due to differences in age distribution; but when this factor is made constant, the divorce rate among the psychotic is still two or three times as great as in the population as a whole.

By far the most complete and the most important study bearing upon the questions here considered, and which is directly relevant to the biological increase of the psychoses, is that of Neil A. Dayton. We present the larger part of his abstract of the scope of his inquiry:

The increasing number of persons with mental disorder requiring hospitalization, and the large numbers involved, draw attention to mental diseases as a major social problem. It is important to know the size of family in this group. Is the stock which produces individuals with mental disorder increasing or decreasing? Our material makes it possible to compare successive generations involving mental disease (Generation I), the number of children ever born to mothers of children later developing a psychosis, and (Generation II) the number of children ever born to married and fecund mental patients. The incomplete families of married and fecund patients admitted to mental hospitals under the age of fifty years are compared with other incomplete family groups. A similar comparison is made for the completed families of patients admitted at the age of fifty years and over. The marital condition of the entire group and the sterility in those ever married are considered.

The material of this communication is based on 15,151 consecutive discharges, including deaths, for the years 1917–28 inclusive, from two large mental hospitals (Boston State Hospital and Worcester State Hospital) in Massachusetts. We have used only one admission of the cases having multiple admissions during this period, and have excluded cases without a psychosis, so that the actual number of patients considered is reduced to 11,959.

We quote Dayton *in extenso:*

We will summarize our data in reference to completed families: (1) It appears that families (Generation I) containing a psychotic individual and families (Generation II) of a psychotic parent (either mother or father) are uniformly smaller than the general run of families in the population of Massachusetts. (2) In the native-born mothers there appears to be no great difference in the size of the two generations; that is, the number of siblings of the patient (Generation I) are practically the same as the number of children born to the psychotic parent (Generation II). (3) When we study the completed families with mother foreign-born, we find approximately the same results. There is a tendency for Generation II to be slightly larger than Generation I.

To have an exact picture of the relative sterility in our social groups, it would be advantageous to compare sterility in Generation II with sterility in Generation I. Insofar as we had no actual figures on Generation I, we were forced to have recourse to sterility in the population at large. This data has been worked out satisfactorily by Lotka. This investigator demonstrated that approximately 17 per cent of all American marriages were childless. We have been forced to use this figure for our comparison. In studying the marriages of psychotic patients we found that 20 per cent were childless. It appeared that the fecundity of an individual (either male or female) married and developing a psychosis after the age of fifty years was lower than that of the general population. Sterility is approximately 3 per cent higher in marriages of individuals with a psychosis than in the general population. Although we may question whether or not sterility is higher in Generation II than in Generation I, we can state that it is unquestionably higher than the general population.

We have seen that the mean number of children ever born to persons developing a mental disorder after the age of fifty is approximately the same as the number born to the parents of these patients and is decidedly smaller than the general population. We have seen, in addition, that sterility in the married psychotics is higher than in the general population. We must now consider the number of our mental patients entering the married state and those remaining single.

A completed family of small size in Generation II plus a higher rate of sterility would be unavailing if a greater proportion of mental patients tended to enter the married state. Considering the large numbers involved, the gross number born would be greater in spite of the observed inhibiting factors. We therefore compared the marital status of our psychotic patients developing a psychosis after the ages of fifty years with the general population of Massachusetts for the same age groups, using the 1920 census as a basis for our rates. The results of these analyses are shown in Chart VII for the males. Taking the married state as a basic rate, we see that approximately three times as many of our patients were single for these age groups as would be expected. The same proportion holds true for the widowed. As we inspect the divorced group we see that this is practically five times that of the married rate. If we inspect the same situation with regard to the females, as outlined in Chart VIII, we see that our curve has essentially the same characteristics. Our material for both sexes indicates that decidedly fewer individuals with a psychosis tend to enter the married state than is observed in the general population.

The reasons for the lower rates in the married group are quite complex. It has been suggested that the economic necessity for family support may keep a number of the married individuals with a psychosis in the community when their mental condition would justify their admission to a hospital for mental diseases, and that the absence of this same necessity contributes to the earlier commitment of the single, widowed, and divorced.

In the married state, either the husband or wife serves as the buffer in protecting the psychotic partner. This protection is effected in two ways: (1) by preventing contact with the outside world and thus concealing the developing symptoms, or (2) by absorbing and minimizing any reactions on the part of individuals who may have had contact with the patient. In these situations the husband or wife is able to protect the partner for some time, and thus produce a decided lag in the commitment of married psychotics.

In the case of widowed or divorced individuals, the factor of protection is lacking, and for that reason their symptoms are observed earlier and their commitment is practically inevitable. In other cases the high rate in the divorced group is due to the influence of mental symptoms which contribute to the family difficulties and result in divorce.

The mental makeup or personal peculiarities of the prepsychotic individual may have made him unattractive to, or not attracted by, the opposite sex, and thus have prevented his entering the married state.

We have seen that Generation II, children of psychotic individuals, is approximately the same size as the preceding generation, but that both generations are decidedly smaller than the general population. We have shown that the marriage rates for our groups are decidedly lower than the general population. To this was added the fact that sterility rates in the married and fecund portion of our patients was decidedly higher than the general population. In addition, a larger proportion of those who do marry become widowed or divorced. The higher rates for dissolution of the family through death or divorce contribute to the small size of family in Generation II by the premature removal of the husband or wife, and thus prevent these families from having their full complement of children. The high proportions of the widowed or divorced also contribute to the high sterility. The high sterility has not been due entirely to this factor, as we found that sterility in the married portion alone was 19 per cent, or 2 per cent higher than in the general population.

Death Rate

When the question of the death rate of the mentally sick and the feebleminded is taken into account, the case for the increase of mental deficiency and mental disease in the population becomes still weaker. Whatever statistical studies have been made strongly indicate the greater morbidity and mortality of the defective and mentally sick groups.

The Metropolitan Life Insurance Company,[1] studying the death rate of the insane in New York state hospitals from 1914 to 1923 and comparing them with the death rates of the same population by sex and age from the years 1919 to 1920, states,

> It is certain that the expectation of life of the insane is greatly curtailed, possibly by as much as one-half. This is obviously a matter of great interest to medical science.

[1] "Mortality of Patients in Hospitals for Mental Diseases"; Statistical Bulletin of the Metropolitan Life Insurance Company, v, 19, no. 5, May, 1928, p. 2.

TABLE V.

Death Rates per 1,000 of the Insane in New York State Hospitals, 1914–1923, Compared with Death Rates of the General Population, 1919–1920. New York State. By Sex and Age.[1]

Sex, Age	Death Rates per 1,000		Ratio of Death Rate of Insane to that of General Population
	Insane	General Population	
Males			
17	53.15	3.95	13.5
22	51.82	5.38	9.6
27	57.05	6.27	9.1
32	72.81	7.39	9.9
37	87.76	8.41	10.4
42	93.87	10.04	9.4
47	95.11	12.69	7.5
52	102.61	17.11	6.0
57	112.04	24.83	4.5
62	137.28	34.35	4.0
67	193.97	50.09	3.9
72	241.67	73.08	3.3
77	356.48	105.93	3.4
82	490.00	156.03	3.1
87	700.00	206.86	3.4
Females			
17	68.79	3.43	20.1
22	80.72	5.28	15.3
27	61.79	6.60	9.4
32	64.81	6.74	9.6
37	59.08	6.73	8.8
42	57.62	8.11	7.1
47	58.86	10.66	5.5
52	67.53	14.40	4.8
57	71.44	21.42	3.3
62	92.07	29.64	3.1
67	129.68	46.70	2.8
72	190.18	69.40	2.7
77	253.61	98.63	2.6
82	355.00	140.30	2.5
87	500.00	199.05	2.5

[1] From the Statistical Bulletin of the Metropolitan Life Insurance Company, 9, 5:2, May, 1928.

It is shown here, for example, that in the age group of males of 17 years, the death rate of the insane is 13.5 times that of the normal population; in the age group of males of 37 years, the death rate is 10.4 times as high as that of the normal population. In the female age group of 17 years, the death rate of the insane is 20.1 times that of the normal population; in the female age group of 22 years it is 15.3 times as high as the normal population. In the age group around 52 years, the difference decreases but is in females still 4.8 times as high as in the normal population; in the males it is 6 times as high as the average population. In the higher age groups the difference becomes still less. In the 82-year group it is 3.1 times as high for males and 2.5 times as high for females than the normal population (Table V.).

Rüdin found that the mortality of schizophrenics as a whole is 3½ (14:4.0417) times higher than that of the mortality of their own normal brothers and sisters, which about corresponds to that of the average population. He claims that this figure represents the true influence of the disease upon the mortality of the afflicted, since other constitutional and conditional factors may be assumed to be the same in this sibling series. In the age group between 21 and 30 the mortality of the schizophrenics is about 5 times as high as that of the normals.

Weinberg, concluding his paper, does not see a great danger in the fertility of the inferior groups, because it is matched by a greater death rate. He also states that the opinions which indicate a great propagation rate of the inferior groups is based on methodologically wrong methods and comparisons.

Meyer, who has made an extensive statistical study on patients suffering from various forms of insanity and epilepsy, found that the mortality of schizophrenics in the age group from 15 to 50 averages 5.4 times that of the average population; that of manic-depressives 15 times; that of epileptics 12 times; and that of the feebleminded twice the mortality of the general population. He states further that of 1,000 people born with a liability to the endogenous mental diseases, only 474 are alive in the age groups from 20 to 50 years, which are the most important for propagation, while of 1,000 normal born persons, 785 reached the age group of 20 to 50 years. This author also doubts that insanity is on the increase and states that nature has barred the endogenous insane from considerable propagation by increased mortality.

EXPECTATION OF LIFE AT AGE 2 YEARS: MALES
(From Dayton.)

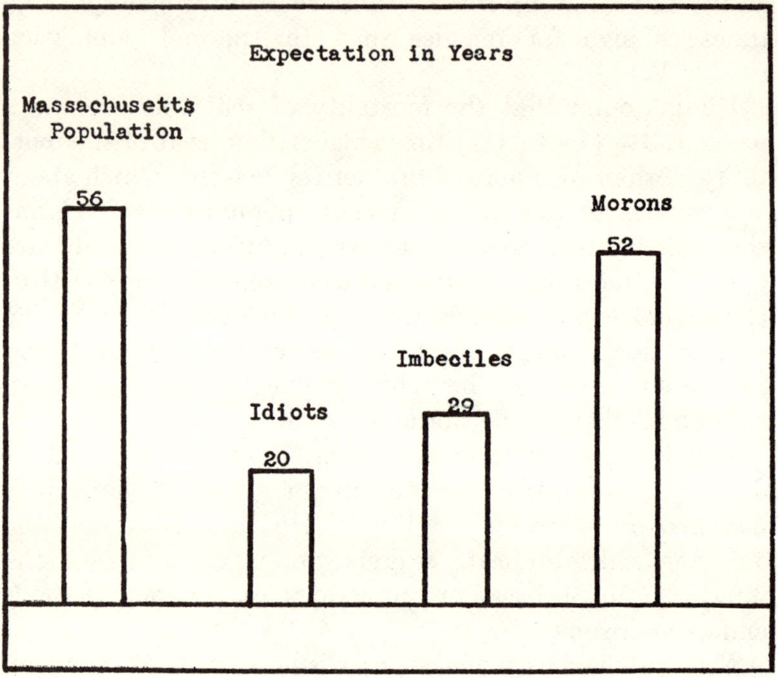

The most thorough piece of work on the mortality of mental deficiency has been done by Neil A. Dayton,[1] who states:

Data on the average expectation of life at certain ages for idiots, imbeciles and morons as compared with the Massachusetts

[1] Dayton, Neil A.: "Mortality in Mental Deficiency Over a Fourteen Year Period: Analysis of 8,976 Cases and 878 Deaths in Massachusetts"; Reprint Proc. of 55th Annual Session of Am. Assoc. for the Study of the Feebleminded, May 25-28, 1931, p. 190.

population show the following results (Table XIX). The average expectation of life for a male infant of two years in the general population is 56.8 years. For idiots this figure is reduced to an average expectation of 20.1 years; for imbeciles, 29.6 years; for morons, 52.2 years; and for mentally defective males as a whole, 30.1 years. For a female infant of two years the average expectation of life is 59.3 years; for idiots, 21.3 years; imbeciles, 38.4 years; morons, 46.8 years; and all mentally defective females, 32.9 years. The average expectation of life for other ages is also presented.

The expectation of life in the presence of idiocy or imbecility is markedly interfered with in each age period. This interference is less marked among the morons, the expectation of life in this group showing only a moderate departure from that of the general population.

Tredgold in his study of 2,219 consecutive deaths in two English institutions emphasizes the fact that "in the mentally deficient the highest death rate falls between the tenth and twentieth years, the period of life in which the mortality rate is lowest among the general population."

LaPage and Barr came to similar conclusions.

The United States Census Report on feebleminded and epileptics in institutions states as follows:

> The death rate among the feebleminded varies in accordance with the degree of mental defect, the general average rates among idiots, imbeciles and morons per 1,000 under treatment being 68.7, 26.7 and 10.1 respectively. The death rate among males in each mental status group is higher than among females. It is noteworthy that this death rate in the moron group approximates the death rate of the general population of the country as a whole.

This brings out the significant fact that there is a decided difference in the number of deaths within each grade of mental defectiveness, and that imbeciles have a death rate comparatively two-and-a-half times that of morons, while the idiots have a death rate nearly seven times that of the morons.

These statements confirm what Myerson has already reported, namely, that taking the cases as a whole, the general bodily physique of the feebleminded shows inferiority in proportion to the amount of feeblemindedness present.

The whole matter of the morbidity of the feebleminded is summarized by Edgar Sydenstricker in the important book "Recent Social Trends in the United States," which is fundamentally made up of reports by former President Hoover's research committee on social trends. "In spite of all efforts to prolong the life of morons, imbeciles, and idiots, they still fail to survive at the same rate as 'normal' persons, especially in the pre-reproductive ages . . . Nature still selects, even though we are horrified by such examples as the Jukes."

We may state, in summarizing the foregoing sections, the following: First, that there is nothing to indicate that mental disease and mental defect are increasing, and from this standpoint there is no evidence of a biological deterioration of the race. What is certain is that hospital population is increasing. The figures from those communities with a sharpened attention to feeblemindedness, mental disease, and epilepsy indicate that where hospital facilities are adequate and where there is a favorable social attitude toward the institutions that there is actually no biological increase in mental disease and, on the other hand, in most of the mental diseases there is either a stationary rate or else a decline. The alarmist attitude is not justified except from the standpoint of the expense of taking care of the mentally sick. To offset this, it is probable that adequate care in the form of adequate institutions acts to remove from the general population the mentally sick and defective and to prevent them from propagating; in other words, that good hospitals and a good hospital system are eugenic measures rather than the reverse.

Furthermore, this conclusion as to the commitment rate is substantiated and perhaps explained by the figures relating to the marriage rate, divorce rate, birth rate and death rate of the mentally sick, diseased, and defective. *Marriage quite evidently is a social factor operating in a eugenic fashion, in that in the case of those who become mentally sick early, the sexual drive is diminished, the capacity for making a living is interfered with, and furthermore, it probably occurs that such people are not attractive to the opposite sex; that their queerness is felt; and that, on the whole, their inferiority breeds a complex of conditions which prevents their marrying.* Even in the case of those who marry, it will be seen that the birth rate is low and the reputedly high fecundity of the mentally defective groups is a myth and based on the assumption that those who are low in the cultural scale are also mentally and biologically defective.

It seems to us, at any rate, established beyond a doubt that the general biological social situations in which the mentally sick and the defective are placed are such as to render precipitate action unnecessary. It does not alter the fact, of course, that sterilization measures have validity if they are effective. Even though there is no increase, the problem is sufficiently great and sufficiently fraught with social disaster and suffering to warrant consideration of this measure as preventive of future mental disease and defect.

We repeat that too much stress has been laid upon *the expense of caring for the mentally sick. That expense is huge but even those communities where state care is low, community care is still considerable although it does not appear upon the official records.* In other words, placing a case of dementia praecox or a case of feeblemindedness in an institution *does not necessarily increase* the cost of caring for him. It may be just as costly to care for him, financially, and more costly from the standpoint of social disorder and familial suffering, in his own home. It is safe to say that when a patient is placed in an institution, the social order is enhanced and that the family can go about their life business with more effectiveness and greater comfort.

In other words, we have no statistics which measure the value of institutional care, the social damage done by keeping the mentally sick and defective in the community. Consequently, the rising cost of the care of the feebleminded and insane is not necessarily a greater cost than where they are not cared for, any more than the hospital population rate reflects a biological increase in mental diseases. We venture to state that *if one adds to the unofficial financial cost of caring for the insane and the feebleminded in the community the unofficial tragedies of arson, murder, and emotional demoralization, the actual cost of institutional care represents financial and human-value economy.*

We shall not consider in detail at this point a further claim of those who are over-eugenically minded that the ameliorative efforts of society keep alive the unfit and act, therefore, as cacogenic measures. This is discussed elsewhere by one of us. If ameliorative efforts did lower the qualities of the race, then we would expect that in those countries where there is a dearth of social effort, the surviving inhabitants would be of finer physique and more resilient mentally than the inhabitants of those countries where social ameliorative measures were conspicuous and part of the organized policy of the community. The Koreans, thus, ought to be finer, stronger, and brighter than the Norwegians, and the inhabitants of some backward American state should present less evidence of deterioration than the inhabitants of Massachusetts. That this is the case needs no refutation at this point. It is precisely in those communities where social care is good that we find the evidence of the finest culture and, on the whole, the best biology. It is in those communities where social care is poor that the population presents an appalling spectacle of degradation.

IV

POINTS OF VIEW REGARDING STERILIZATION

We have sufficiently indicated that there is a very strong movement, especially in the United States and in Germany, for sterilization. The laws represent a more or less moderate attitude, certainly in respect to their enforcement. That there are those who would go far beyond anything at present established as legal is quite evident in the literature. Thus, Whitney, one of the leading writers in eugenics, believes that about one-tenth of the population should be sterilized. Furthermore, certain enthusiastic proponents of eugenics have formulated what is called an "ideal" sterilization law which has been considered of sufficient validity by them as to be proposed for legislation. This "ideal" sterilization law sets up an enormous group of conditions, some of which are clearly environmental, as requiring sterilization on the ground that the individuals are socially inadequate persons, and it further "establishes" as cacogenic the individuals who, whether or not they show any defect, and whether or not their immediate descendants show defect will "by the established laws of heredity be the probable potential parent of socially inadequate offspring."

Elsewhere Myerson [1] has criticized this proposal and we need not consider it further at this point except to say that while there seems to be no immediate danger of this pro-

[1] Myerson, A.: "A Critique of Proposed 'Ideal' Sterilization Legislation"; Arch. of Neur. and Psychiat., Mar. 1935, v. 33, 453.

posed law being enacted, those who are friendly to eugenics and those who value human liberty and individuality ought to take a very firm stand against such over-dogmatic and socially excessive measures.

As an example of this point of view, Fritz Lenz, one of the leading Germans in the entire field, states:

> Sterilizations on this small scale (referring to those in the United States) are obviously insufficient for a real purification of the race. A race hygiene commission under the leadership of Laughlin has developed quite a radical program, under which almost 1/10 of all living people would be sterilized. In the first year, approximately about 100,000 sterilizations should be performed, increasing up to about 400,000 in 1980 at which time about 15,000,000 inferior people would be sterilized. The whole bulk of inferior people should be either segregated in institutions or sterilized. People who remain permanently in institutions should not be sterilized. Inmates who have recovered and from whom only inferior progeny could be expected should be discharged if they are sterilized. One cannot deny that the execution of such a far-reaching program would essentially contribute to the well-being of the race, but at this time it would not be practical even in the United States.

The Catholic Point of View

We now turn to one of the leading forces against sterilization, namely, the Roman Catholic Church. The position of the Catholic church is definitely set forth in the encyclical of the present Pope:

> Finally, that pernicious practice must be condemned which closely touches upon the natural right of man to enter matrimony but affects also in a real way the welfare of the offspring. For there are some who over-solicitous for the cause of eugenics, not only give salutary counsel for more certainly procuring the strength and health of the future child—which, indeed, is not contrary to right reason—but put eugenics before aims of a higher order, and by public authority wish to prevent from marrying all those whom, even though naturally fit for marriage, they consider, according to the norms and conjectures of their in-

vestigations, would, through hereditary transmission, bring forth defective offspring. And more, they wish to legislate to deprive these of that natural faculty by medical action despite their unwillingness; and this they do not propose as an infliction of grave punishment under the authority of the state for a crime committed, nor to prevent future crimes by guilty persons, but against every right and good they wish the civil authority to arrogate to itself a power over a faculty which it never had and can never legitimately possess.

Those who act in this way are at fault in losing sight of the fact that the family is more sacred than the State and that men are begotten not for the earth and for time, but for Heaven and eternity. Although often these individuals are to be dissuaded from entering into matrimony, certainly it is wrong to brand men with the stigma of crime because they contract marriage, on the ground that, despite the fact that they are in every respect capable of matrimony, they will give birth only to defective children, even though they use all care and diligence.

Public magistrates have no direct power over the bodies of their subjects; therefore, where no crime has taken place and there is no cause present for grave punishment, they can never directly harm, or tamper with the integrity of the body, either for the reasons of eugenics or for any other reason. St. Thomas teaches this when, inquiring whether human judges for the sake of preventing future evils can inflict punishment, he admits that the power indeed exists as regards certain other forms of evil, but justly and properly denies it as regards the maiming of the body. "No one who is guiltless may be punished by a human tribunal either by flogging to death, or mutilation, or by beating."

Furthermore, Christian doctrine establishes, and the light of human reason makes it most clear, that private individuals have no other power over the members of their bodies than that which pertains to their natural ends; and they are not free to destroy or mutilate their members, or in any other way render themselves unfit for their natural functions, except when no other provision can be made for the good of the whole body.

Moreover, the leading Catholic theologians and biologists, and we may here cite as exemplifying this group Mayer, have always been skeptical, from a scientific point of view, of the validity of sterilization, despite the fact that Mayer has been quoted as friendly to sterilization by Popenoe.

Mayer's principles in respect to sterilization deserve quoting. He believes that there is an increase in the insane, criminal, and feebleminded. He discusses the possibilities of expulsion, isolation, and sterilization. His studies bring him to the following conclusions:

1. Certain hereditary insane and criminals can only produce inferior children. Consequently, and because they cannot properly educate their children, they may lose their right of propagation.
2. An inferior progeny may be a danger to the state. In this case the state should have the right to protect itself by inhibiting procreation.
3. One of the measures that is to be considered is sterilization. This should only be considered, however, as a last remedy if all other measures are inadequate or impossible. Its applicability should be considered from two angles—first, from a matter of principle, and second, from a practical point of view.
4. Principal conclusion: Since this question is still open theologically for discussion (this was written before the encyclical of the pope which ends the discussion), causes pro and con can be discussed. Theoretically, the principle can be established as sententia probabilis that legal sterilization of the mentally diseased is not bad in itself, because it aims at a good goal with good will, but it is only then ethically permitted and good in itself if its necessity for the commonweal raises it into the sphere of the ethically good. Therefore, a need for society must be existent, and it must be proven without doubt that this need is brought about by the procreation of the mentally diseased and by the constant qualitative diminution of the hereditary endowment of the people which leads to the deterioration of the commonweal. Furthermore, before such a measure can be established, the heredity of mental disease and its damaging influence upon the commonweal must be scientifically proven. Finally, it must be actually practicable, and it must achieve its aim, namely, the salvation and protection of society.

Mayer goes on to state:

The survey of these data leads us to the conclusion that legal sterilization in our countries today will have to be denied for practical and social ethical reasons. The following facts are definite:

1. Up to date the conditions for legal sterilization are lacking, since

a. No European state can prove that its existence and well-being is endangered by an over-large birth rate of the hereditary mentally diseased and criminals.

b. The science of heredity today is definitely not in a position to make in any specific case a definite diagnosis or even probable prognosis of heredity. Futhermore, it is an established fact that the degeneration of society is more related to extrinsic (environmental) damage than to intrinsic hereditary causes. Society, therefore, has the duty to establish social and moral reforms for avoiding this kind of degeneracy by education, social measures, assistance to those who are willing to procreate and, if necessary, should also resort to legal compulsory measures against the obvious moral and social irresponsibility prevalent in the circles of the intellectuals.

He goes on to state:

We have emphasized and demonstrated that legal sterilization in our present state of knowledge would not be able to achieve its aim, because medicine has no reliable and useful methods of sterilization (sic). In the present primitive state of genealogic research very few judgments could be safely passed, and the scanty success of such judgments would not be in any reasonable proportion to the necessary effort.

Mayer ends up this particular section with the statement:

The whole historic development of the sterilization of the mentally sick and the general interest demonstrates sufficiently that here we have to deal with a very serious problem. The question is still more serious because medicine and psychiatry are just at the beginning and not at the end of the field of psychiatry and social hygiene. Therefore, the conclusion can be reached from this entire book that practically speaking a legal sterilization of the mentally sick at the present time would be premature, useless, and unworkable, and therefore, from a practical point of view prohibitive and morally objectionable.

That not only the Catholics but that many sociologists

are opposed to sterilization is exemplified by the writings of Charles A. Ellwood, who states:

> It is a counsel of perfection, which modern science has given us in the doctrines of eugenics; but like all such counsels it is socially valuable and is obviously closely allied with idealistic social religion. If eugenics were ever made the basis of a code of minute legislative prescriptions regarding marriage and reproduction, doubtless it would become an intolerable tyranny. But, as the basis for social ideals regarding marriage and the birth of children, it is invaluable. Social religion, not less than eugenics, is interested in securing wise marriages and in making sure that every child is well born. Social religion, too, should emphasize the social service which parents render to society in the birth and rearing of normal children. . . . It will make the birth of children in the family welcome in proportion as there is health and strength and economic means to give them a fair start in life, and it will condemn the selfish individualism which shirks the obligations of parenthood. Finally, it will seek to create in the young a eugenic conscience which will safeguard marriage and the birth of children. Only thus can the ideals of eugenics stand any chance of realization, as Sir Francis Galton, the founder of the movement, himself recognized. Here again we see the essential identity of interest of applied social science and social religion.

In a very eloquent passage Hobhouse states substantially this—that eugenics postulates that we know what is *eu* and that we also know the *genics* of the situation. He states that in both these respects we are decidedly deficient. The time has not yet come for a program based on our rudimentary knowledge.

Most of the English biologists are quite skeptical of sterilization. Thus, Professor A. V. Hill states that if we could prevent parenthood among all mentally defectives, we should on some assumption reduce their numbers in the next generation; but if repeated in the next generation, it would have comparatively little effect.

Professor Punnett indicates that it would take between two and three thousand years to reduce the incidence of mental defect to one in 10,000. This is probably to be classed as a scientific guess.

Henry Herd, the psychiatrist, states that no general measure of compulsory sterilization is justified, first of all, because of our ignorance of the method of transmission of the mental defect; and secondly, even assuming Mendelian transmission, by our inability to detect the carrier. "It is literally true to say that we do not know who should be sterilized in order to eliminate the defective. Only a voluntary measure of sterilization can be at the present time justified, but it is mere self-deception to believe that sterilization is in any way going to reduce the matter of the incidence of deficiency."

The British, on the whole, are moderately in favor of voluntary sterilization. A comprehensive study is the report of the Departmental Committee on Sterilization, which was published in December, 1933 as an official document of the British government. On this board were the following members: L. G. Brock (chairman); Wilfred Trotter; R. A. Fisher; A. F. Tredgold; Miss Ruth Darwin; E. W. Adams; R. H. Crowley; and E. O. Lewis to be a committee "To examine and report on the information already available regarding the hereditary transmission and other causes of mental disorder and deficiency; to consider the value of sterilization as a preventive measure having regard to its physical, psychological, and social effects and to the experience of legislation in other countries permitting it; and to suggest what further inquiries might usefully be undertaken in this connection." (This discussion will be cited in a later part of our report.)

The general headings include preliminary general considerations as to legal position, concept of mental defect, the extent of the problem, present knowledge of the causation of mental defect, the influence of environment and its relation to heredity, and certain general conclusions on the causation of mental defect, which we will discuss later. The

Commission goes on to the causation of mental disorders, studies the results of sterilization both socially and biologically, considers the legislation on the matter, and as a result of the entire study concludes that they "were impressed by the dead weight of social inefficiency and individual misery which is entailed by the existence of over one-quarter of a million mental defectives and of a far larger number of persons who, without being certifiably defective are mentally subnormal. This mass of defectives and subnormals is being steadily recruited and is probably growing. . . . We were increasingly impressed by the injustice of refusing to those who have good grounds for believing they may transmit mental defect or disorder and who are in every way unfitted for parenthood the only effective means of escaping from a burden which they have every reason to dread."

Their summary of practical recommendations follows:

1. Subject to the safeguards proposed, voluntary sterilization should be legalized in the case of:—

a. A person who is mentally defective or who has suffered from mental disorder;

b. A person who suffers from, or is believed to be a carrier of, a grave physical disability which has been shown to be transmissible; and

c. A person who is believed to be likely to transmit mental disorder or defect.

2. Before sterilization is sanctioned in the case of a mental defective, care should be taken to test his or her fitness for community care.

3. Mental defectives who have been sterilized should receive the supervision which their mental condition requires.

4. The operation of sterilization should only be performed under the written authorization of the Minister of Health; in regard to which the following procedure should apply:—

a. Application for the authorization should be supported by recommendations in a prescribed form signed by two medical practitioners, one of whom should, if possible, be the patient's family doctor and the other a practitioner on a list approved by the Minister. No medical practitioner should sign a recommendation unless he has examined the patient.

b. The Minister, on receipt of the recommendations, should be empowered to require any necessary amendment of the forms and to cause the patient to be especially examined if it is considered advisable.

c. In order to deal with difficulties that may arise in connection with applications on behalf of persons suffering from, or believed to be carriers of, inherited disease or disability, the Minister should be empowered to appoint a small advisory committee consisting partly of medical practitioners and partly of geneticists to whom doubtful cases could be referred.

d. The hospital authorities or (in the case of operations performed elsewhere) the operating surgeon should be required to notify the Minister when the operation has been performed.

e. In all cases in which the patient is capable of giving consent, he should sign a declaration of willingness to be sterilized, and one of the two medical recommendations should include a statement that the effect of the operation has been explained to the patient and that in the medical practitioner's opinion he is capable of understanding it. If the practitioner is not satisfied that the patient is competent to give a reasonable consent, the full consent and understanding of the parent or guardian should be obtained. If the applicant is married, he or she should be required to notify the spouse of the application.

f. In the case of persons who have suffered from mental disorder, sterilization should not be permitted without a recommendation from a competent psychiatrist, who should be required to certify, after examining the patient, that, in his opinion, no injurious results are likely to follow.

g. In dealing with cases of mental defect and of mental disorder, the Minister of Health should exercise his functions after consulting the Board of Control.

h. The procedure should at all stages be treated as strictly confidential.

5. Medical practitioners, in making recommendations for sterilization should have protection similar to that accorded to them in respect of certificates given under the Lunacy and Mental Treatment Acts.

6. The operations for sterilization which are recommended are vasectomy in the case of males and salpingectomy in the case of females. The latter operation should only be performed by a

surgeon competent to deal with any morbid condition which he may find.

7. The operation of vasectomy should not be authorized in the case of any person who has not reached physical maturity, pending the results of the research recommended in this connection.

8. The operation for sterilization should not be performed in a mental hospital or mental deficiency institution.

9. In the case of persons unable to pay the full cost of the operation, the cost (including the expense of the medical recommendations) should be borne by the Mental Deficiency Authority in the case of mental defectives, by the Visiting Committee in the case of persons suffering from mental disorder, and by the Public Health Committee in the case of persons suffering from transmissible physical disorders, subject to the right of the authority to recover from the patients or relatives so much of the cost as is reasonable. In all cases, however, where the cost falls upon local funds, the local authority should have the right to require the patient to enter a municipal hospital or any voluntary hospital with which they may have made arrangements for such cases.

10. In addition to the research mentioned (in 7) above, further recommendations for research are made in Chapter VII which do not permit of presentation in a summarized form.

In 1930 in order to obtain the opinion of the total members of the American Association for the Study of the Feebleminded, a questionnaire was sent to the 317 members. This was followed up by a second questionnaire and by April 30, 1930 replies were received from 258 members, representing 80% of the total membership. The general opinion of this important group was this: 94% of the replies received favored sterilization; 97% of these voted for selective sterilization, non-compulsory. The opinion was that heredity has been overemphasized and that emphasis in sterilization should be laid upon the term selective rather than eugenic.

V

GENETICS AND ITS RELATION TO EUGENICS

ON THE whole, eugenics receives scant support on any scientific basis from genetics. Genetics has largely concerned itself in the past twenty-five years with those experimental procedures by which, in lower animals especially, the genes have been discovered and their laws of appearance and combination have been formulated. The literature on this subject is vast and hugely important to mankind, but as yet fundamentally inapplicable to those situations with which this committee is concerned. In order for a character to be studied genetically, it must be susceptible of experimentation, that is, it must be clearly defined; and second, breeding experiments are essential. In this way, the fruit-fly and its characters have been thoroughly investigated, and there has developed an actual geography of the localization of the genes in the chromosomes which represents the ingenuity and the triumph of scientific men in the highest degree. But the characters of the fruit-fly and, for example, dementia praecox in the human being stand in different planes of scientific thought and approximation. The generations of the fruit-fly rapidly succeed one another. The environment can be controlled, and the scientist acts as the *deus ex machina* of the whole life of the experimental animal. One need not go into detail to contrast this situation and that surrounding dementia praecox to any group of neurologists and psychiatrists, or to any thinking persons.

Furthermore, in order for a character to be susceptible to

genetic understanding at the present time, it must, in some measure at least, become established as Mendelian. We will show later that this is not the case in any complete way in any of the psychoses, mental deficiency or epilepsy. It is true that many men have set up the hypothesis of Mendelian recessiveness of one type or another in the case of the conditions we are studying. But nothing like proof has been adduced. The leading geneticists, at least of America and England, have been very cautious in their pronunciamentos concerning eugenics, and it is apparent from their writings that they look with disfavor upon the sweeping statements made popularly and, to some extent, in the scientific literature concerning eugenic measures.

Morgan states:

The inheritance of derangements of the mental faculties of man is a very difficult problem, partly because there are few, if any, parallels in other animals that can be experimentally tested, partly because the diagnosis in man is often uncertain, and partly because the environment is a complicating agency. . . .

At the other extreme is human intelligence, man's most valuable asset. Is intelligence inherited? There is a widespread belief that it is, and I should be far from wishing to gainsay it. The main difficulty is one of definition. It is commonly assumed that there is one, and only one, criterion of intelligence—that we are speaking always of the same thing when we use the word. In reality our ideas are vague on the subject . . . But this averaging of many heterogeneous things has in the past often led to very erroneous conclusions. So far as heredity is concerned, it is a procedure that the majority of geneticists avoid if possible. Accurate work in heredity can only be attained when the diagnosis of the elements of a situation is known. . . . The difficulty, of course, is—aside from our inability to define what is meant by intelligence—that we do not know here how much is due to nature and how much to nurture. . . .

For example: genetics has taught us how congenital malformations can be most quickly eliminated from the germinal material, or at least reduced. On the other hand, it is obvious that wise human conventions will not permit any such extremely drastic treatment as this procedure might suggest to the fanaticallyminded uplifter. The doctrine that all men are born equal carries with it the assumption that they be allowed to breed as they will.

Morgan further states, warningly,

It is conceivable that when man undertakes to direct the evolution of his race, he may blunder badly.

Such remarks as these of Morgan may be multiplied by the statements of Jennings, Castle, Haldane, and many others. It is true that the geneticists believe that the race can be benefited enormously by good breeding and by the elimination of undesirable stocks, but they are, on the whole, not convinced that mankind knows enough about the mental diseases and the effects of the social structure to manipulate in a successful way the procreation of the race.

Moreover, it is clearly becoming apparent that geneticists and biologists, generally speaking, are retreating from the position in which they were placed by a whole-hearted acceptance of Weismannism. The reaction against Lamarck was extreme. It became quite the biological fashion to deny the environment any place in the constitution of man, despite the obvious fact that nowhere in the world is there a germplasm which is not continually being bombarded, penetrated, and continuously molded by the environment. Germplasm is no abstract substance and neither are the genes. Both are bathed in the internal environment of the living creature which harbors them, which means the blood containing gases, food-stuffs, living organisms of infectious or other type, and coming down to more subtle matters—radioactive substances. In fact, the whole cosmos in one form or another, as it enters the living body, is in chemical and physical interaction with germplasm and gene.

Apart from this generalization, the facts as they have developed have shown conclusively that for the genetic substance to express itself as a character, a set of environmental circumstances of a stable type are necessary. That which comes down as a set of hereditary characters operating according to the Mendelian law under certain thermometric and barometric conditions in a laboratory entirely disappears and is replaced by a new set of characters under radically changed thermometric and barometric conditions. It is definitely established that by focusing the environment upon the germplasm, thus upon the genes, the mutation rate is enormously increased.

If we make a formulation of heredity which will involve the present known facts, we can state as follows: we may conceive of the hereditary substance lined up in parallel rows of genes with specific qualities for each group of genes and the appearance of characteristics in the progeny according to the Mendelian laws, as they express the more or less random shuffling of the genes during the process of germ cell maturation and the subsequent recombination of the genes at the union between the male and female gametes. This, however, does not express the entire genetic relationship. There are other factors which are of genetic importance:

First, *the environment may be conceived of as a releasing agent for the manifestation of a character without which, so to speak, the character could not appear*. Thus, in the study of genetics in drosophila, the following characters have been shown to be directly affected in their expression by the environment:

Number of teeth on the sexcomb (unfavorable environment decreases number).

Longevity (affected by crowding and temperature).

Vestigial wing (high temperature increases length).

Abnormal abdomen (most pronounced in moist cultures, almost disappears in dry environment).

Reduplicated legs (most pronounced and higher percentage affected at low temperatures).

Bent, rough eyes, abnormal bristles (affected by low temperatures).

Abdominal spotting (temperature affects the number of abdominal spots).

Variable eye (most extreme in warm dry conditions).

We may mention the darkening effect which cold temperature has upon the expression of certain members of the albino series in laboratory mammals.

A number of inherited characters are known whose presence would never be suspected were it not for the specialized artificial environments provided by modern scientific techniques. Among such characters we may include the A-B type of blood groups of many mammals including man, hyperglycemia in mice, and a lack of complement in guinea-pigs.

The allergies also afford examples of genetic characters whose presence is often unsuspected until some specific factor in the environment elicits the reaction which characterizes them. Thus, if no pollen is in the air a man may never suspect that he inherited the gene for hay fever. Thus, a Mid-Westerner who never eats fish does not suspect that he has an inherited sensitivity to fish. Thus, thousands of persons do not know that they are by genetic constitution sensitive to the emanations of horses, rabbits, canaries, primroses, strawberries, and many other agents unknown to their intimate environment.

These examples will suffice to show that many genetic characters remain latent, unless developed or made manifest by some specific factor in the environment.

Second, we have to consider *what has been styled the residual heredity or the intra-genetic environment*. There is now on record a considerable body of evidence to show that often a few and sometimes many genes in the residual hereditary background of an individual affect the expression of a single gene being studied. An example is that of the rodless retina in the mouse which normally possesses one row of external nuclei. During experiments with this character there arose intermediate types, some possessing about three rows of external nuclei, and others about six rows, probably due to selection of modifiers or the residual heredity of the animal.

It is a common experience in dealing with mouse spottings for example to come upon the effects of modifying factors. In other words, some genes augment one another; on the other hand, some genes causing similar effects do not augment each other. In laboratory animals and frequently in man, we find hereditary characters which are not "good dominants"; others are not "good recessives." They fluctuate quantitatively. Such characters may be called "irregular dominants." Regarding recessive characters, it may be stated that some are incomplete and are so styled "incomplete recessives," as when head-dot in the mouse, which is ordinarily recessive, may occasionally produce hybrid animals bearing a few white hairs on the forehead, but which transmit the character in the ordinary recessive fashion.

In the minds of these who have studied such fluctuating characters, there is little doubt but that this fluctuation is due to modifying factors in the residual heredity of the individual, factors so numerous and in their individual effects so minute that they escape individual identification. It is also apparent from drosophila studies that if a gene moves to a new neighborhood within the chromosomes through the processes of translocation or inversion that the character it produces is in some cases altered. This fact demonstrates that a gene interacts with and its effects may be modified by the nature of its immediately neighboring genes.

Quantitativeness of the Gene

While most geneticists believe that the strength of a gene is constant and that fluctuations and expressions in different individuals, such as we have just described, are due at least in the cases examined to other genetic and environmental fluctuations, it is not probable that this expresses the entire state of affairs.

Timoféeff-Ressovsky shows that the genetics of Drosophila funebris are somewhat different from the genetics of the fly usually studied (Drosophila melanogaster), and that variations in character arise which seem to be due to the "penetrance" quality. This practically means that for any genetic substance like a gene, there is both quality and quantity which can be altered by external factors such as low temperature, etc.

Plate, also, states that the gene is not constant.

Blastophoria

Medical men have for a long time laid emphasis on what is known as blastophoria, by which they mean to imply that the genetic substances are susceptible to injury and will transmit injured individuals; in other words, the genetic substance may suffer from disease as may any other part of the body. This concept is called blastophoria and was introduced by August Forel. This view is not shared, however, by the experimental geneticist.

Adami stated as follows years ago:

> To the worker in bacteriology the hesitance on the part of biologists to accept environment as a most important factor in originating variation is almost incomprehensible. . . .

Adami would have rejoiced in the experiments of Hoffmann who increased the mutation rate enormously by the use of X-rays and gave a most important impetus to the concept that the environment is in intimate relationship with the germplasm in all its manifestations. He states the following:

> No, in the first place, we have clear evidence that the germ cells are not, after the Weismannian conception (as usually accepted), so sacrosanct that they are insusceptible to influences which affect the body at large. Even though their growth is restricted still they have to grow, and they have to maintain existence, and growing they must absorb and assimilate material brought to them by the blood and diffusing from the blood into the lymph. If that lymph contains soluble toxic substances, the germ cells are not precluded from absorbing them as do the other cells of the body—and, like those other cells, from being influenced by them. I have brought these examples forward on previous occasions, and they have never been rebutted; on the contrary, the evidence of this order is steadily increasing.

The experiments on blastophoria have, on the whole, suffered from the fact that diverse interpretations may be made of the results. Elsewhere, one of us has cited a good deal of the literature on the subject.

Nor must we forget there is one important environment in man's history which as yet has not been studied and that is the uterine environment. The first and most plastic period of life is spent there. What happens there is still unknown. Hogben, for example, states that the importance of the intra-uterine environment is indicated by the high incidence of malformation in children born of mothers approaching the menopause.

That there may be genetic poisons which alter the quality of the genes so that impaired and defective individuals appear in a hereditary manner is a concept that need not be dismissed cavalierly. *Negative results are only applicable to the experiments which produce them.* It is interesting in this relationship to note that one of Hoffmann's earlier papers indicated that the environment could not produce mutations, yet it was only a few years later, by using another technique, that he produced an enormous increase in the mutation rate.

We may present as the newer attitude of biology and genetics the following exposition of Riddle's beliefs based on his own work and the experimental genetics:

The real nature and role of heredity is much misunderstood. Moreover, it is usually so described as to place in a false and inferior light some of the most significant advances being made in other branches of biological research. . . . It has become clear that the specific *conditions* under which a gene or factor operates and develops have an equal value with the germinal factors in the appearance of anything that can be called heredity. The factors distributed by germ cells set limits to the nature and appearance of adult characteristics. So do conditions. To use the recent apt words of Jennings (1925), "The characteristics of the adult are no more present in the germ cells than are those of an automobile in the metallic ores out of which it is ultimately manufactured. To get the complete, normally acting organism, the proper materials are essential; but equally essential is it that they should interact properly with each other and with other things. *And the way they interact and what they produce depends on the conditions.*"

He then goes on to state:

Heredity is controlled whenever and wherever an aspect of development is controlled.

Riddle gives specific instances, such as the classic experiments on the salamander, on stature, and on gigantism. He further states, "In some lower organisms it has been found possible to change or to reverse the basic pattern—the polarity—of the organism"; and that sexuality can be changed or reversed by the experimenter. He then goes on to give an example of controlled heredity in man in the clinical observation that melanin distribution in the skin becomes changed under the conditions of nerve injury; sexual maturity and immaturity in animals can be, in large measure, controlled by the use of endocrinal injections. Moreover, he cites instances where the germplasm itself was modified as in the experiments of Harrison and the work of Muller.

Space forbids us to give Riddle's own experiments on the relationship of the endocrine glands to reproduction and the enormous change which can be made in the development and general biological pattern by the manipulation of the endocrines. His whole thesis, which seems to us to be extremely pertinent to the problems of psychiatry, is that by manipulating both the external environment and the internal environment of the individual that, first, the characters of the individual may be altered from their otherwise normal hereditary pattern; more importantly, that there is work to show that the germplasm itself may be modified.

Constitution

Although the concept is as ancient as Hippocrates, a great deal of stress has been laid in modern literature on what is known as constitution. By general usage the term means in pathology a liability to disease in a quantitative relationship. For example, some people have a greater liability to infection by the tubercle bacillus than others, owing to a congenital or inborn lack of resistance factors. Thus, there is a diabetic constitution, and similarly with the liability to arteriosclerosis and cardiac disease. In psychiatry the concept has been amplified in recent times so that certain psychiatric types are really constitutional types, such as is found in the division of mankind by Kretschmer and others. It is common now to speak of the schizoid type or the cyclothymic type. The usual implication that this is necessarily hereditary, however, is in certain measure fallacious. On this point we quote Raymond Pearl:

> It (referring to his concept of constitution) implies that while a man's constitution is relatively stable because heredity plays a great part in its determination, it is not something absolutely

constant throughout his life. On the contrary, on this view, the constitution of an individual at any given moment is in part the resultant of his past history—the diseases he has had, the vicissitudes of embryonic development through which he passed, and so on.

The evidence that a man's biological constitution may change fundamentally during his lifetime is abundant and convincing. Consider, for example, a man who has smallpox in his thirties, and recovers from the illness. He may go on living until he is ninety. But during this long period he is immune to smallpox. He may make intimate contact with the most virulent cases of active smallpox and suffer no harm. As a result of having had the disease once he has, as an individual, undergone a profound and irreversible alteration of his biological make-up. And if this specific immunity so acquired is not to be thought of as properly a part of his constitution it would seem best to stop talking about constitution at all. If an individual were known to be born with such a complete immunity to smallpox (as presumably some people are) no one would hesitate to call it a truly constitutional peculiarity of that individual. What warrant biologically is there for regarding it as less so when it is acquired? I know of none.

And Pearl, after citing the work of the experimental embryologists, states:

In sum, an individual's constitution is what he *is*, the totality of his particular individual being biologically considered, without particular immediate concern as to how it came to be what it is.

The environmental events which may change constitution are not limited by clinical experience to infection, although the more striking cases occur after the circumstances of infection. Thus, the remarkable change in personality which follows encephalitis may definitely be called a psychic constitutional change on a physical basis. The post-traumatic constitution, described by Meyer, which is so common in clinical experience is a remarkable instance of this same constitutional alteration through environmental events. While it may be that the bulk of constitutional abnormality which psychiatrists deal with may be inherent, there is nothing definitely to prove this to be the case in any total sense.[1]

[1] For further references in this connection see Myerson, A.: "The Inheritance of Mental Diseases"; Williams & Wilkins Co., Baltimore, 1925, p. 127.

VI

STUDIES ON THE INHERITANCE OF MENTAL DISEASES

IN THE following section we discuss the heredity of schizophrenia, manic-depressive psychosis, feeblemindedness, epilepsy, and crime, more or less as if these were definable entities, and thus that it is possible to study them statistically and scientifically. No psychiatrist of first rank believes this to be the case; for him the term dementia praecox, for example, represents the best we can do in the way of classifying what is obviously a group of conditions which is very likely of heterogeneous composition. Thus, the differences in diagnosis between neighboring institutions, *concerning the same cases,* may be so great as to plunge the psychiatrist into despair and the scientific observer of any designation into something like contempt.[1] In whatever degree these conditions are not entities in that degree the conclusions regarding their inheritance are invalid. But we cannot go ahead of present day knowledge, and we may properly, although cautiously, consider the situation even as it exists today.

[1] See in this connection the comments in Myerson, A.: "The Inheritance of Mental Diseases"; Williams & Wilkins Co., Baltimore, 1925; pp. 264 ff. See also the following papers in "Schizophrenia, Statistical Studies from the Boston Psychopathic Hospital, 1925–1934: Elkind, Henry B.: "The Application of Statistical Method to the Study of Mental Disease"; Doering, Carl R. and Raymond, Alice F.: "Reliability of Observation in Psychiatric and Related Characteristics"; and "Additional Note on Reliability."

1. Polymorphism

It is necessary, in order to consider the validity of conclusions to examine, first of all, the technique by which the data upon which the conclusions are based have been obtained, and often this brings us, first of all, to the underlying theory which directs the research. Most of the work done in the heredity of the psychoses has its logical, almost its philosophical sanction, in the theory of polymorphism. This generalization may be summed up as follows:

There is a unitary something, in the neuropathic and psychopathic inheritance, which makes itself manifest under many forms (thus, the polymorphism). All manner of mental disease, including the organic mental diseases, are thus labeled, and all psychoses, including feeblemindedness, epilepsy, and crime. Up to this day this doctrine governs in most of the studies made of the heredity of mental disease and appears under a new guise in the Mendelian work. It has been given the sanction of the foremost writers until very lately. In the excessive development given this theory, headache in an ancestor was given a hereditary value in relation to the mental disease of his descendants. Fainting spells even in a cousin had a dread significance, and the early writers laid great stress on tuberculosis, cancer, hemiplegia, gout, "rheumatism" and every chronic or semichronic human ailment.

Lombroso and his pupil Nordau gave to the term degeneracy, which is merely a synonym for polymorphism, its widest significance, so that on the one side cretins, idiots, etc., were linked together in a hereditary chain with the men and women of genius on the other. Their "reasoning" is typical of that of the whole polymorphic school, including the writings of Morel, Féré, Déjérine, Clouston, MacPherson, Barrett, and others. Lombroso based much of his theory on his idea of the stigmata of degeneracy which are both physical and mental. Thus, he gives as the signs of degeneracy common to both genius and insanity shortness, tallness, rickets, lameness, hunched back, pallor, emaciation, stammering, left-handedness, delayed development, precocity, and includes such matters as "fondness for certain words".

In Féré's "La famille neuropathique" is as typical an account of polymorphism as is found in the literature. What may be called clinical blurring is found at its best in his pages, although others than clinicians have linked together convulsions, hysteria, idiocy, epilepsy, strabismus, paralysis, neuralgia, cerebral inflammation, deaf mutism, exophthalmic goiter, gout, and paralysis agitans, as neuropathic. Thus, a similar polymorphism forms the basis of the results and conclusions reached by Davenport in his earlier studies on the heredity of mental diseases, and especially the heredity of epilepsy.

It is obvious that to disprove or prove polymorphism, it would be necessary to carry on extensive studies of the heredity of the normal population or, at least to avoid the word normal, that part of the population which is not labeled insane, feebleminded, epileptic, criminalistic, and degenerate. Such control studies have appeared only sporadically in the literature, and none has been large enough.

Wagner von Jauregg's remarks in respect to the polymorphic theory are pertinent and of great value. This distinguished psychiatrist states:

> Pedigrees have been gathered in which mental and nervous diseases, suicide, etc., in brief, all those characters which are considered as taints, have been found in many members of the family. This method is of some use for didactic purposes, but as proof it is worthless. No matter how many tainting factors may appear in a pedigree, this may always be the result of chance. If I put all numbers from 0 to 9 in a bag, and draw a number four times in succession, it is very improbable that I shall draw number 9 four times in succession; but in 10,000 cases this will occur once in accordance with the laws of chance. But those only are chosen from among the pedigrees in whom severe tainting has been expressed; it would be a simple thing to contrast these with

a large number of pedigrees in which only isolated taints occur, or none at all.

In this connection we may quote Pollock and his coworkers:

> The sample of the insane is drawn from a comparatively small population. Thus, a sample of the insane in New York would be drawn from a hospital population of 50,000. A corresponding sample of the non-insane would be drawn, however, from a population of over 12,000,000. Consequently, if we choose equal samples of the two groups the possibility of random variations is decidedly greater in the sample drawn from the larger population. Both samples should be similar in all respects to the populations from which they are drawn. This means that the sample must have the same composition with respect to sex, age, race, social constitution and other important characteristics, as the universe of individuals from whom it was selected. Clearly the larger the population from which the sample is drawn, and the more complicated its make-up, the more difficult will it be to make the sample truly representative.

It may be stated that practically no comparative study has kept in mind these important considerations and that, consequently, we have very little real information upon which to base any far-flung theory of the heredity of the psychoses or of feeblemindedness. Thus, in the classically quoted work of Brugger only 117 normal control families were used, a number entirely insufficient. Luxenburger and Schulz studied only 182 families of the population of Munich, which is certainly a small sample.[1]

While the work of Koller and Diem was based on insufficient numbers and the conclusions impaired by the fact that the normal were younger people than the insane, and furthermore all types of insanity were lumped together, it appears from their work that the sane have more nervous

[1] There is such marked divergence in the results obtained by Brugger in Basel and Luxenburger and Schulz in Munich as to confirm the belief that the samples were far too small for any statistically valid conclusions.

disease, apoplexy, and senile dementia in their heredity and through their collateral ancestors than do the insane.

Jolly, studying 200 normal and 200 mentally sick, shows that the total hereditary taint in the old sense, that is, in the polymorphic sense, is not much different in the sane than in the case of the insane. The mentally sick, however, show a great deal more of mental disease in the ancestry than do the normal; while, on the other hand, organic nervous diseases, apoplexy, and the functional nervous diseases are more common in the ancestry and relatives of the normal than those of the abnormal. Thus, any research which gives weight to these latter factors in the psychoses is invalidated in the measure of the weight given.

The difficulties of forming conclusions concerning polymorphism may well be exemplified by Stein's excellent paper on epilepsy. He compared the family histories of his 1,000 patients at the Monson State Hospital for Epileptics with a somewhat larger number of histories obtained from non-epileptic individuals who themselves had never had a seizure. The two groups are, in the first place, very definitely dissimilar in constitution. The institutionalized patients at Monson represent the lower stratum of the population, meaning by that people who are more exposed to sickness, bad environmental conditions, accidents, injuries and all the things that go with the poorer conditions of life. The controls are physicians, social workers, medical students, teachers, etc., obviously on the whole a more favored group. Moreover, the family histories in the case of the institutionalized group were taken by physicians directly from the relatives and were supplemented by investigation by social workers in the community. The family histories of the non-institutionalized group were taken by a questionnaire method which, from the standpoint of the time given to the case and the accuracy of the results, was probably much less valid than the histories of the epileptics.

Let us compare, for example, the incidence of migraine in

Stein's group of epileptics and his group of controls with its incidence in certain other groups. Stein finds a history of migraine in 17% of the immediate families, including parents, siblings, and children, and in a slightly lower percentage of the control group. Cobb, studying a group of 100 non-institutional and non-traumatic cases of epilepsy, finds an incidence of 4.3% of migraine in the family history. Burr entirely omits migraine from his study of epilepsy on the grounds that it is one of the commonest of diseases. Patrick and Levy find the frequency of periodic headache in groups of apparently normal women in five communities as high as 40.2%, and consider even this figure probably too low. Migraine has been considered an important "neuropathic trait" especially in the heredity of epilepsy, but in the face of these figures, and the fact that people who have the one disease rarely have the other, the foundation for such a belief may be seriously questioned.

Similarly with the incidence of mental disease. In the relatives of the epileptics, Stein finds a higher percentage of mental disease than in those of the normal group (0.4%), but Pollock, discussing Stein's paper, remarks that the amount of mental disease in the controls was much less than that usually found in the "total population" which is 4.5%; whereas among parents, siblings, and children of Stein's normals, only 0.4% was found. It is obvious that his was an unusual group, highly selected and probably not of the same age as the epileptic group.

Moreover, when all mental diseases are linked together under the term "psychoses" and all feebleminded under the heading "feeblemindedness," the results must be definitely erroneous. It has been shown by all the recent workers that there are only two psychoses which have a hereditary significance of importance—manic-depressive and dementia praecox. Dividing up the feebleminded into definite groups, Myerson and his co-workers state that the sporadic cretins, Mongolians, and organic brain cases have no especial relationship to heredity, so far as this can be discovered by the study of family histories. It is only in the group in which no organic or pathological explanation can be found that inheritance appears as an important factor.

We may also discuss the case of alcoholism as a polymorphic and hereditary etiological factor in the production of mental disease. We find very curious contrasts in the results obtained. Thus, if one takes the studies of Elderton and Pearson on alcoholics in Scotland, and contrasts them with the studies made by Rüdin in the ancestry of the schizophrenics, the results are almost imcomprehensibly different. Elderton and Pearson found that, on the whole, the descendants of the alcoholics were physically better off and showed no more incidence of mental deficiency or mental abnormality than the descendants of the non-alcoholic! But Rüdin, disregarding this, has given weight to alcohol as a factor in the production of dementia praecox (see section on dementia praecox). Even in the case of his work, the number of families has been, on the whole, insufficient for scientific conclusions. It is relevant to say that while Rüdin is a cautious polymorphist, his general trend is away from polymorphism.

Canavan, studying 581 children of non-psychotic parents and contrasting them with the 463 children of dementia praecox stock comes to the following conclusions: The backward and nervous are equal in numbers in the offspring of the dementia praecox and the non-psychotic parents. The cases of conduct disorder are higher among children of the psychotic, nearly five times as much, perhaps because of the lack of home control. But there are more cases of physical disease in the offspring of the non-psychotic parents, although the death rate is lower. There were more feebleminded in the offspring of the normal parents, ten of them being feebleminded, whereas there were only four among the offspring of the praecox parents. In other words, so far as Canavan's material went, feeblemindedness certainly had less relationship to dementia praecox than to normality.

The analysis of the cases of Krueger, Luther, Schlub, Riebeth, and Myerson indicates definitely that the psychoses of brothers and sisters tend, on the whole, to be alike, at least in the main characters. Throughout the literature the more careful case studies indicate definitely that manic-depressive insanity and dementia praecox do not tend to occur in the same stock. Furthermore, the psychoses of parents and children, although differing somewhat in the main take the same general trends. And Beck finds an interesting similarity between the patterns of even the symptomatic psychoses expressed by parents and children.

While a certain possible trend toward polymorphism may be found and while it is possible that the constitution which develops, let us say, epilepsy has some relationship to the constitution which develops dementia praecox, the relationship is not close enough to warrant the postulate of any widespreading unitary trait back of all psychoses, feeblemindedness, epilepsy, and the like. Consequently, a great deal of the work which has been done is entirely invalid and has only historical significance. This applies quite decidedly to such work as is exemplified by the study of the publicized feebleminded families, the Nams, the Kallikaks, the Jukes, and such types. It invalidates, we believe, the earlier work which comes from Davenport, Rosanoff, and the American Eugenic school with its headquarters at Cold Spring Harbor, New York. We may fairly state that the eugenic studies of Lombroso, Morel, Esquirol, and others should now be relegated to the history of psychiatry rather than to its actively utilizable material.

This is the conclusion reached by Genil-Perrin as the result of an exhaustive study of the history and the effect of the theory of mental degeneration, and which deserves a wider recognition than it has received. He disposes of the whole polymorphic doctrine as follows: The doctrine of mental degeneration constitutes one of the most important facts in the evolution of psychiatry but it is time that it entered into the domain of past history!

2. Studies on Specific Mental Diseases

We now come to the discussion of the heredity of the specific psychoses. It may be stated at once that while there may be a constitution which develops general paresis, none has been proven, and we may regard this disease as exogenous and outside of the realm of our discussion. At this point, however, it is pertinent to remark that the term *constitution* and the concept, while very valuable and useful for medicine, has been decidedly over-worked. It is obvious on a logical basis that no one can get a disease for which he has no predisposing constitution. If the human-being were entirely insusceptible to tuberculosis, as some animals are, he could not be infected by the germ. If skulls were made of sheet-iron, a falling brick would be fractured rather than the skull. The fact that the skull is bone gives it a constitution which predisposes it to fracture. Nevertheless, from the practical standpoint, the skull would not fracture by itself, and it is the impact of the falling brick which, in a naïve sense, causes the fracture of the skull.

We may also exclude from our discussion the alcoholic psychoses—without alcohol, no alcoholic psychosis; just as has been stated—without syphilis, no paresis. The problem of mankind in relationship to the alcoholic psychoses is fundamentally this—either through education, or legislation, or both, to bring about temperance or abstinence in the use of alcoholic beverages.

Nor need we consider the senile dementias and the arteriosclerotic psychoses. These are hugely important in their numbers and in the burden they impose on the state, but by no conceivable method could we discover a way of anticipating their incidence. Furthermore, the individuals who have these psychoses have usually lived normal and useful lives and as yet no one is hardy enough to suggest that we sterilize to prevent psychoses occurring beyond the age of 55, and usually in the sixties. In fact, to get a senile psychosis is a mark of biological vigor, since it indicates that the patient has been able to survive the vicissitudes of life into old age. Furthermore, the probable difference between the person who acquires senile dementia and the one who does not, both being senile, is quantitative. Probably any person who lived long enough would develop a dementia, and the diseases of senium are too closely allied to the normal conditions of senility to be discussed in any hereditary or preventive terms in the present state of our knowledge.

We also exclude from our consideration such diseases as pellagra. Davenport made a gallant effort to link up pellagra with heredity, but modern science has definitely shown that this is a disease of the vitamin deficiency group, and can be both prevented and cured by proper diet and general hygienic conditions. Similarly, with the rarer psychoses, such as those associated with organic brain disease, such as brain tumor, multiple sclerosis, Parkinson's disease, and the like. The cases are few; they are substantially problems of the diseases of the nervous system, for which no clear-cut heredity of any kind has been postulated in the literature, although cases do occur which indicate that a similar constitution among siblings brings about these diseases.

We turn, therefore, to the two important psychoses which are linked up with heredity—schizophrenia and manic-depressive psychosis; and to feeblemindedness and epilepsy.

a. Schizophrenia

The first study of the inheritance of schizophrenia to be carried out on a large scale was that of Lundborg, who studied the occurrence of the disease in a group of families totaling 2,232 members in the rural province of Blekinge in Sweden. He found that in this group dementia praecox and related forms of psychopathy appeared in proportions which comes close to those he believed one would expect in a recessive type of inheritance. In some of Lundborg's families myoclonic epilepsy was also endemic.

Wittermann subjected his families of schizophrenia to a quantitative Mendelian analysis and stated that his figures corresponded with those which one would obtain if dementia praecox were a simple recessive Mendelian character.

Rosanoff added to the statements of Lundborg and Wittermann his concept of allelomorphic heredity of schizophrenia and believed, without any real demonstration, that epilepsy, dementia praecox, manic-depressive psychosis, imbecility, involutional melancholia, paranoid psychosis, acute alcoholic hallucinosis, and similar mental diseases stand in a hereditary relationship to one another, these psychoses being recessive in varying degrees, while mental health is dominant. The sequence of recessivity would be from the dominant normality to manic-depressive insanity, dementia praecox, and epilepsy. Thus, he sets up an allelomorphism of mental disease and normality.

Oberholzer considers schizophrenia to be a recessive character and bases this conclusion, to some extent, on the fact that the indirect inheritance of dementia praecox, that is, from an uncle, aunt, or collateral to the patient, and especially the occurrence of dementia praecox among siblings, far outweighs the direct heredity from parent to child.

Rüdin, in his celebrated studies, found direct heredity extremely rare. Studying more than a thousand families of Kraepelin's clinic in Munich, he found 34 cases in which parents and children were suffering from dementia praecox.

We now propose to examine in more detail the situation in respect to dementia praecox, and especially the proposition which assumes that there is a Mendelian character operating to bring it about. We shall consider in some detail the statistical method which has been used and the correction which Weinberg, Levy and others introduced and which completely overturned the concept previously held. The most important material has been gathered by Rüdin and, practically speaking, the work done by Rüdin, Hoffmann, and Luxenburger constitute the only studies which were comprehensive enough to be of real value, if we exclude from the present consideration the work on monozygotic twins. In the discussion we shall use the term *propositus,* which is a translation of the German word *proband,* to mean the individual patient around whom the heredity study has been developed.

It was the achievement of Weinberg, to have demonstrated conclusively that the results of Wittermann, Lundborg and Rosanoff on schizophrenia, as well as the work of Davenport and Weeks on epilepsy, and other work on inherited disease were mere statistical illusions due to the artificial elements of selection. These authors selected cases in which at least one diseased person already existed, namely, the propositus, and counted him as well as the other cases found in the family history. In this way, as Weinberg demonstrated, the investigators studied only those products of DR x DR crossings which had resulted in at least one diseased, but this is only a part of the total possibility of results, even according to the strictest Mendelian laws.

By plotting the probability of offspring from DR x DR crossings, assuming that a large number of families may have two children each, the following 16 combinations are possible: in one case, both children may be recessively diseased homozygotes, and these will both manifest dementia praecox. In two families one individual of each family will represent a recessive diseased homozygote, presenting, for example, dementia praecox, and one dominant healthy homozygote. In four families, of the two individuals of each family, one will be a recessive diseased homozygote presenting the disease, and the other will be obviously healthy (phenotypically healthy), but will be a heterozygote. There will be nine families in which no case of dementia praecox will appear, of which four will present phenotypically healthy but genotypically heterozygotic groups. Four other of the families of these nine will be obviously healthy, one member of each being a pure dominant healthy one, the other member of these four being phenotypically healthy but a heterozygote recessive. The last of the nine families in whom no case of mental disease will be found will be dominant healthy. This, of course, is for two children family groups. When families of four or more children are postulated, that is, of a size large enough for Mendelian ratios, the variety of genetic types becomes exceedingly complicated.

The workers whom Weinberg has criticized have studied only the seven cases in which dementia praecox appears and have found the probable recessive statistical ratio, but it is obvious they should have studied as well the nine other families, including eighteen individuals who present no cases of mental disease. Thus, these workers should have found instead of 25%, 57.14% cases of dementia praecox in the selected sub-group. Consequently, it appears from their own statistics that dementia praecox is certainly not a pure recessive character, since the quantitativeness of its occurrence is too small to warrant those conclusions.

To avoid this artifact of statistics, Weinberg devised his new method of statistical approach called by him the "Probanden methode," which essentially excludes the selected propositi from the count.

On the whole, his method, although it has some errors (see Bernstein), gives roughly valid results. The effect of the application of Weinberg's principles is quite startling. Rüdin has subjected his figures to a pre-Weinbergian as well as a Weinbergian analysis. According to the old method, the percentage of the incidence of schizophrenia among siblings of schizophrenics would be 24.67%, a figure which comes quite close to an "ideal Mendelian" ratio. By applying Weinberg's method, the incidence is only 4.48%, which is less than 1/5 of the expected ratio. This illustrates the difficulties of heredity studies, since by simply using another statistical method, the results differ as 24.67% differs from 4.48%.

Rüdin's results, which we have cited above, were carried out on a series of 701 families with 4,823 siblings, of whom 765 were schizophrenics. As stated above, the results gave an incidence of 4.48%, but by using an abbreviated method of calculation, the incidence is 5.35%. Rüdin states that other non-schizophrenic psychoses occurred in this group in a proportion of 4.12%. Discussing these results, Rüdin concludes that schizophrenia cannot be a simple recessive Mendelian character, otherwise 25% of the brothers and sisters of schizophrenics would also be diseased. He offers, therefore, a hypothesis of two complementary characters, both of which must be present to produce schizophrenia, both being recessive, while two other dominants determine the result free from schizophrenia. However, such a dihybrid recessive inheritance would require a proportion of 6.25% of incidence among the siblings of schizophrenics, and this figure is not reached in his cases.

Rüdin discusses the possibility of relating schizoid psychopathic personalities to schizophrenia but he is aware of the danger of thus widening the definition of schizophrenia, "until no man finally may be called free from it."

The conclusion of Rüdin that dementia praecox represents a set of dihybrid recessive characters can be criticized on the ground that he has assumed something which cannot be proven, and the possibilities of such an inheritance and its manifold crossings are almost impossible to calculate in the human being. Moreover, he has followed Weinberg's rule which essentially is deducted from a pure recessive mode of inheritance, while he himself is in favor of a dihybrid one. We feel that no conclusion is justified from his results other than to state that in his group of siblings one out of 22 was also afflicted.

A further chapter in Rüdin's book deals with the incidence of schizophrenia among the offspring of one schizophrenic and one phenotypically healthy parent, who have one schizophrenic child. The series was collected directly from patients in the psychiatric clinic in Munich, in which a diagnosis was established by direct study. Only 34 families of this type were found in Rüdin's material, and there were altogether 166 children, or 4.88 children per family. In this group of siblings, 37 *including the propositi* were schizophrenics, that is to say, 3 in addition to the patients themselves. Besides this, 18 other families from other hospitals had been selected by Rüdin, totaling 22 schizophrenic children, but these have not been included in the statistical study. Thus, of the brothers and sisters of a schizophrenic child who has one schizophrenic parent, Rüdin states 6.18% are also suffering from schizophrenia, that is, less than one out of 16. But other non-schizophrenic psychoses in this group occurred in a percentage of 10.30.

It may be objected at once that after all Rüdin only found three more schizophrenics than he started with; that this number is not sufficient to establish any rules or regulations or any calculations of a valid type which establishes a Mendelian ratio. The only conclusion justified from this part of Rüdin's study is that in a particularly narrow selected group, schizophrenia occurred in three additional cases. The figures come from a highly selected group, since there must be, and there are definitely known to be, schizophrenic parents who have no schizophrenic children, and thus the percentage of 6.18 is definitely too high to be representative of the proportion of schizophrenia in the offspring of schizophrenic parents as a whole. Whatever the cause of schizophrenia may be, whether due to the unfavorable combination of parental genes, or due to environmental influences on some underlying condition, no Mendelian hypothesis on the basis of Rüdin's figures seems justified. Moreover, Rüdin has made a simple statistical error in reaching the conclusion of 6.18%. Excluding the propositi, there were 3 additional schizophrenics among the 132 siblings of these 34 individuals. The proportion of 3 to 132 is not 6.18%; it happens that it is only 2.27%. On the whole, one may state, on the basis of Rüdin's cases, that the presence of a schizophrenic parent among the ancestors of a schizophrenic patient does not greatly increase the risk of schizophrenic descendants within the limits of ordinary probable error of calculation.

At this point it is relevant to consider Hoffmann's data. Like Rüdin he has collected cases of schizophrenia occurring where the parents were not schizophrenic and found in his material of 20 families a total number of 20 schizophrenics among 88 siblings. He calls this an incidence of 22.7%, but the critical observer will note that actually not even a single schizophrenic has been added by him to his propositi. In other words, he commits the error which Weinberg so trenchantly criticized. In a second series of 4 families, he found 5 schizophrenics among a total number of 15 siblings. Thus, he added one to the total number of propositi and this by selecting from the total number of material in Tübingen; and concludes there is an incidence of 33.3% schizophrenics. Under such circumstances, obviously the number of cases is altogether too small for any conclusions.

Rüdin further takes up the problem of the relationship of other conditions to the incidence of schizophrenics. Thus, the occurrence of another non-schizophrenic psychosis in one parent results in a percentage of 8.21 dementia praecox among the siblings; in other words, the astonishing result is found that dementia praecox on this basis is more related to other psychoses than to dementia praecox itself. Further, when another group is taken, where both parents were suffering from some mental disease other than dementia praecox, it will be found that 22.72% of the siblings were suffering from dementia praecox. This group is made up of 10 families with 59 siblings. A third group concerns the siblings of cases of dementia praecox whose parents were alcoholic but who were not suffering from any mental disease. Here it was found that 7.80% of the siblings had dementia praecox, the material being made up of 109 families with 784 siblings. The most astonishing result is obtained in his fifth group which consists of those siblings of schizophrenic parents, the parents of whom are free from dementia praecox and other mental disease, but in whose families some remote collateral incidence of dementia praecox had occurred. In this group, dementia praecox occurred in 8.07%, the material consisting of 62 families with 421 siblings. Thus, it would seem to be eugenically better to have a schizophrenic or alcoholic parent than to have two healthy parents and some remote collateral occurrence of schizophrenia.

To show the strange conclusions which may be drawn from such statistical studies as Rüdin's, it is noteworthy that step-siblings of schizophrenics have an incidence of schizophrenia which is only 0.56% and therefore lower than the average population. This mathematical result was derived from 134 families having 498 siblings. This would seem to indicate that it was eugenically good for a normal person to mate with a person who has already had schizophrenic progeny by a previous mating.

The criticism that can be made of all this work is that there were no control studies, an elementary scientific need. For example, no control study has been made of the results of alcoholism in the general non-hospital population. Similarly, no control study was made as to the incidence of dementia praecox in cases where there were two healthy parents and dementia praecox occurred in some collateral or side line, but with no patient in the hospital. Rüdin has selected his material in a way which, in the last analysis, destroys his conclusion, that dementia praecox is a recessive character of dihybrid origin, for if we accept all his conclusions in relationship to dementia praecox, we must

TABLE VI.

Survey of the Percentage of the Frequency of Schizophrenia in Children According to Status of Parents

Groups	Exact Calculation			Abbreviated Calculation			No. of Families	Total No. of Siblings
	Schizo-phrenia	Other Psychoses	All Psychoses Together	Schizo-phrenia	Other Psychoses	All Psychoses Together		
I. Both parents free from schizophrenia DR x DR crossings	4.48	4.12	8.6	5.35	.....	.....	701	4823
II. One parent schizophrenic: RR x DR crossings				6.18	10.30	16.49	34	166
III. Step-siblings				0.56	1.70	2.27	134	498
IV. One parent suffering from some insanity other than schizophrenia with or without alcoholism of one or both parents				8.21	8.21	16.43	133	881
V. One or both parents suffering from insanity other than schizophrenia, and one or both parents alcoholic				14.81	7.40	22.22	36	244
VI. One parent alcoholic, neither parent mentally diseased				7.80	5.20	13.01	109	784
VII. Both parents suffering from mental disease other than schizophrenia, with or without alcoholism				22.72	.....	22.72	10	59
VIII. Propositi tainted with schizophrenia in collateral side lines. Both parents free from schizophrenia, alcoholism, and other mental disease				8.07	6.83	14.90	62	421
IX. One parent suffering from insanity other than schizophrenia and one or both parents alcoholic				15.78	7.89	23.68	33	223

(From E. Rüdin: "Studien ueber Vererbung und Entstehung geistiger Störungen"; Monog. a.d. Gesamtgebiete der Neurol. u. Psych., 12, 1916, p. 73.

conclude that alcoholism also is a form of dementia praecox or contains within it those genes which lead to dementia praecox. We may also have to conclude that normality is the same thing. Rüdin has been too selective both of his material and of his results.

Barrett, who is a frank believer in polymorphism, has made a study based on 150 consecutive admissions of schizophrenics at Ann Arbor. He cites Kraepelin who found that in 1,054 cases of schizophrenia mental abnormalities and factors commonly considered as of importance in genetic relations in the psychoses occurred in a percentage of 68.3 among their families. He also cites Bleuler, who, basing his figures on Wolfsohn, gives a hereditary tainting of 90%.

Barrett used the controls of Koller and Diem for normals; those of Kalb for paresis; those of Snell for epilepsy, and those of Sünner for manic-depressive psychosis.

As hereditary tainting factors, Barrett accepts the psychoses, and includes feeblemindedness, epilepsy, and the psychoneuroses, suicide, abnormal character, nervous diseases, alcoholism, and apoplexy. His conclusions are:

> In a series of 150 unselected cases of schizophrenia there were 117, or 78.01% that had heredity tainting factors, usually considered as of significance in the heredity of the psychoses. *This is about equal to that found for psychoses in general and considerably greater than that of the non-psychotic,* 78.01:67. (Italics our own.)

This does not seem to us to be markedly greater in view of the number of factors which are considered of significance and the relatively small number of cases.

> It is slightly less than has been found in manic-depressive psychoses, 78.01:84.13% and in epilepsy, 78.01:81.26. The most frequent tainting factor is the psychoses. These occur among the mental abnormalities of the antecedents and members of the families in a percentage of 43.22. (It is to be remembered that this term psychoses includes as well epilepsy, feeblemindedness, and the psychoneuroses.)

This is about three times greater than has been found in those who are not psychotic.

The difference between the normals and Barrett's schizophrenics in relationship certainly to the total hereditary taint, is not significant if we take into account the small number of cases of the normal population which has been studied and also the small number of schizophrenics. When the psychoneuroses are included as a hereditary tainting factor, it would seem inevitable that a population of sufficient size be surveyed for the incidence of this condition. It has been stated that the psychoneuroses probably constitute the most common illness that mankind has with the exception perhaps of the "cold." We are not convinced that this approach to the heredity of dementia praecox is a valid one, and certainly nothing in Barrett's own figures proves that dementia praecox is an inherited character of complex

TABLE VII.

Hereditary Tainting in 150 Cases of Schizophrenia*
(Only the nearest tainting factor counted)

150 cases of schizophrenia (Barrett)	Direct		Atavistic	Collateral	Siblings	Total	Percentage					
							Direct		Atavistic	Collateral	Siblings	
	Father	Mother					Father	Mother				
Psychoses.....	11	11	10	13	4	49	7.33	7.33	6.67	8.67	2.67	32.67
Nervous diseases	2	...	2	...	...	4	1.33	.....	1.33	.....	....	2.66
Alcoholism.....	14	...	4	1	...	19	9.33	.....	2.67	.67	....	12.67
Apoplexy......	1	...	14	2	...	17	.67	.....	9.33	1.33	....	11.33
Senile dementia.	...	...	1	...	...	1	.....	.....	.67	.....	....	.67
Abnormal character.......	9	4	3	6	3	25	6.	2.67	2.	4.	2.	16.67
Suicide.........	...	...	1	1	...	2	.....	.....	.67	.67	....	1.34
Total........	37	15	35	23	7	117	24.66	10.	23.34	15.34	4.67	78.01

* (From Barrett, Albert M.: "Heredity Relations in Schizophrenia"; Am. Jr. of Psychiatry, v. 7, 1927–1928, p. 78.)

Mendelian type, unless it be assumed that alcoholism, epilepsy, the psychoneuroses, feeblemindedness, abnormal character, and all of the mental diseases are part of this complex Mendelian character. The term *Mendelian* has merely been substituted for *deviation from normality* in the widest possible sense, and all of its value as a precise method of studying heredity has been thrown overboard.

In the average population, if one plots together Luxenburger's and Schulz' material in Munich, schizophrenia occurs in a percentage of 0.85. The material of Luxenburger and Schulz together consists of 695 individuals out of 182 families. The propositi of Luxenburger's material have been gathered from healthy spouses of general paretics. Brugger, in Basel, studied 452 individuals out of 117 families, the propositi being spouses of paretics, tabetics, brain tumor cases, and other organic nervous diseases. In this population he found an incidence of schizophrenia of 1.53%. He concludes from this study that the incidence of schizophrenia in Switzerland is higher due to the decrease of exogamy. He also found that suicide in Basel is 4.2 times as frequent as in Munich, and emigration is 3.6 times as frequent.

Adding to the material of Brugger, Luxenburger and Schulz that gathered by Kattentidt and Göppel, a group of the average population of altogether 4,127 people is available. Among this group schizophrenia occurred in 0.75%. It should, however, be stated that Kattentidt's material includes 270 cases, who also have been used by Luxenburger and, therefore, are reduplicated. The actual amount of the material therefore is 3,857 cases.

An important paper is that of Pollock, Malzberg, and Fuller, which is abstracted as follows:

The study of causative factors in dementia praecox may begin appropriately with an analysis of the family stock of such patients. Because of the difficulty of finding specific environmental or exogenous factors adequate to account for the origin and development of the disorder, there has been a tendency to favor the viewpoint of heredity. Such an interpretation must find its basis in the investigation of the frequency of mental disorders among the relatives of patients with dementia praecox. Logically, of course, the existence of several cases of a disease within a family is not conclusive proof of inheritance, for environmental factors may have caused them all, as in the case of typhoid infection. On the other hand, the absence of exceptional frequencies of mental disease within a family stock, must be interpreted as proof of the lack of a hereditary basis. For this reason it is essential to clear the ground by beginning with a survey of the family stock.

The basic material of this study consists of the family histories of 175 patients with dementia praecox received at the Utica State Hospital during the three years 1928 to 1930, inclusive. No selection was exercised in the choice of patients, other than the existence of a well-defined psychosis. The histories were gathered from the testimony of the patient, the relatives and other interested and informed individuals. Wherever possible, the authenticity and accuracy of the data were checked by social workers, both at the hospital and in the field. (For a more detailed description of the method and fields of investigation, see Psychiatric Quarterly, v. 8, no. 1, p. 77–78.)

Of the 175 patients, 92 were males and 83 females, a ratio of 110.8 males to 100 females. This is a close approximation to the sex ratio among all first admissions with dementia praecox to the New York civil state hospitals. (Forty-fifth Annual Report of the New York State Dept. of Mental Hygiene, p. 192.) It differs significantly from the sex ratio among first admissions with manic-depressive psychoses. In the latter group in this period females predominate among first admissions in the ratio of 157.0 females to 100 males.

Summary: In the families of the 175 probands with dementia praecox there was an expectation of 94.6 cases of mental disease, based upon the general expectations in the state of New York. The 'corrected' total of cases was 121.5, which exceeded the expected total by 28.4%. The excess is even more significant, when it is recalled that the 'corrected' total is only a minimum, and that, were the histories of the older generations more detailed, the total of mentally diseased would probably be increased.

Among the siblings of the probands the information is undoubtedly more reliable than in the older degrees of relation. Among the brothers there was a 'corrected' total of cases of mental disease of 23.7, compared with an expectation of only 15. Among the sisters the 'corrected' total was 22.4, compared with an expectation of 12.0.

There appears to be a tendency for relatively more tainting in the relatives of the male probands. In view of the small total, however, the results can only be considered suggestive. Thus among the siblings of the male probands, there was an excess of 86.6% of the corrected total of mentally diseased over the expected total, whereas among the siblings of the female probands the corresponding excess was only 55.1%. Whatever interpretations one may attach to such differences, they are surely significant when contrasted with the corresponding results in the families of the probands with manic-depressive psychoses. Among the latter there is clearly more tainting in the families of the female probands, and more tainting among the female siblings than among the males. (Psychiatric Quarterly, v. 8, no. 1, p. 96-97.)

The siblings of the probands with dementia praecox show greater frequencies of dementia praecox than are expected on the basis of general expectations.

It must therefore be concluded that there is a greater probability of mental disease among the relatives of patients with dementia praecox than exists in the general population of the state of New York. Unless there may be discovered other specific factors capable of explaining the appearance of mental disease in these families, it must be assumed that family predisposition is an important etiological factor.

The discrepancy between the actual total and the expected Mendelian total is still too great to be explained away. Among the 329 siblings still alive and more than 15 years of age at the time of the investigation, we should expect a total of 82.3 $\pm$ 5.3 tainted individuals. The lower limit of expected cases may be put at 66, compared with 20 actual cases. In order to bring the total up to Mendelian expectations, it would be necessary to develop at least 46 additional cases in this group during the remaining life of the generation. This would indicate an expectation of mental disease of almost 15 per 100, which is in overwhelming excess over the general expectation at the same ages, and consequently exceedingly improbable. We must, therefore, conclude that the statistics of mental diseases in these families are not consistent with a Mendelian explanation.

In another group of 47 families, one parent was classified as DR, there being no outward evidence of a mental disorder. The other parent was assumed to be of the Type of RR, being described as alcoholic or nervous. In such matings, half of the offspring should be tainted (RR) and the other half outwardly normal but latent bearers (DR). The statistical data are summarized in Table VIII.

TABLE VIII

Offspring of Parents of Assumed Type DR x RR, Classified by Age at Death, or Age at Time of Admission of the Proband to the Utica State Hospital (from Pollock, Malzberg and Fuller).

Age (years)	Deceased Siblings*		Living Siblings*	
	No. of Cases	Number with Mental Disorder	No. of Cases	Number with Mental Disorder
Under 10	29		2	
10–14	2		7	
15–19	3		16	1 dementia praecox
20–24	3		18	1 manic-depressive 1 nervous
25–29	1		22	1 dementia praecox 2 nervous
30–34	1		16	1 dementia praecox 1 alcoholic 2 nervous
35–39	2		16	1 manic-depressive
40–44	..		10	1 nervous
45–49	2		4	
50–54	2	1 alcoholic	4	1 nervous
55–59	..		3	1 nervous
60–64	..		1	
65–69	1	1 with cerebral arteriosclerosis	..	
70–74	..		..	
Total	46	2	119	14

(*Exclusive of proband)

It is evident that tainting factors in the parents, such as alcoholism or nervousness, are associated with a higher frequency of tainted offspring. Thus in the preceding matings, the tainted offspring represents $9.7 \pm 1.6\%$ of the total offspring. Among the 458 offspring of the outwardly normal parents, the percentage of tainting among the offspring was only 5.7 $\pm$ 0.73. The difference, however, is less than 3 times its probable error, and therefore cannot be regarded as statistically significant.

It is clear, therefore, that though there is probably a familial basis for the origin of many cases of mental disorder in the family stock of probands with dementia praecox, the observed frequency cannot be described in Mendelian terminology.

It should be noted that those methods which enable us to classify the parental generations in plants and animals in Mendelian terminology, are largely inapplicable in the case of man, and the genotypes representing dominance among the latter are, therefore, a matter of supposition rather than of observation. This uncertainty in the parental generation clearly affects the validity of the interpretations of the filial generation. In the second place, as pointed out by Bleuler (Mendelismus bei Psychosen, speziell bei Schizophrenie. Schweiz. Arch. Neur. 1. 1917, p. 35), there is grave doubt that we are dealing with a unitary disease in the case of dementia praecox, and it is entirely possible that the etiology may differ in the several types. Furthermore, there is reason for believing that environmental agencies affect the origin and course of the disease, and thereby influence the totals of affected offspring. The fact that the latter are so much less than the totals required by Mendelian theory point to the probability, that although inheritance plays a general role in the transmission of these diseases, environmental influences nevertheless are also important factors.

The committee believes it may be stated in reference to the role of the environment in the case of dementia praecox that the citing of "positive instances," as the authors do, where some environmental event is related to the onset of dementia praecox is, in the last analysis, totally unprovable and at the present time distinctly unscientific. It may be and there probably are environmental factors connected with the onset of mental diseases, but candor requires one to say that neither worry, social strain, sexual difficulty, trauma or any other happening can be classed as more than coincidental. In view of the frequency of distribution of these events in the lives of the general population, it is yet to be proven that they occur more significantly in the case of the patients with mental disease than in the case of the people of the general population. Trauma, for example, is far more frequent in the history of men than of women, but there is no difference of incidence of dementia praecox which corresponds at all with the difference of incidence of this factor.

Other miscellaneous studies of some importance are here listed:

Luxenburger found that among siblings of his Munich dementia praecox material, the psychosis had an incidence of 5.0%; while Brugger found the percentage to be 10.7 in Basel. Nieces and nephews of schizophrenics have a disease incidence of 1.4% according to Schulz, while Brugger's figures are 3.5%. Juda, studying grandchildren of patients with dementia praecox in Munich gives the incidence as 1.8%, while in Basel the same worker finds a percentage of 4.0. This may show a diminishing tendency in the remoter generation.

In a study of the occurrence of schizophrenia among the ruling houses of Europe which he considers one large family with schizophrenic recessive tainting, all being direct descendants of Charles of Valois and Margaret of Naples, his second cousin, Luxenburger comes to the conclusion that schizophrenia has a tendency to crop up where inbreeding or unsuitable exogamy (marriage between two tainted families) occurs, while it is avoided by suitable out-breeding. Luxenburger thinks that schizophrenia is a complicated recessive character, very widespread in humanity, which may crop out in any social or racial group that limits its exogamy by exclusiveness and therefore may be apt to be found in inbred aristocratic families as well as those of the ruling houses.

Leo Alexander studied a large family with a high incidence of schizophrenia, residing in one village for seven generations. After two perfectly healthy generations, inbreeding takes place in several instances and schizophrenia crops up here and there; however, it disappears in a number of branches after out-breeding takes place again.

In spite of the criticism we have made of the above material, it is probable that there is some hereditary factor operating in the production of dementia praecox, although it cannot be stated that this has been satisfactorily demonstrated in a clear-cut, incontrovertible way. To call it Mendelian one has to go through that type of mental gymnastics particularly prevalent where a thesis has to be proven. How potent that hereditary factor is, in what percentage it operates certainly is not known. It may be even greater in potency than appears in Rüdin's figures, for it often happens that a person who is normal at one period of study turns out to be dementia praecox ten years later. Therefore, it is probable that dementia praecox occurs in certain families in a higher incidence than in the general population. This, we believe, is about the only definite statement which can be made at the present time.

b. *Manic-Depressive Psychosis*

It is curious to note that while the literature is quite unanimous as to the hereditary character of manic-depressive psychosis, very little valuable statistical material is available. Many authors present only charts of selected and particularly highly tainted families. The group has been somewhat widened since Kretschmer's publications, since he also included the hyperthymic and depressive temperaments into the manic-depressive psychoses and classified both the traditional manic-depressive cycle and the cyclothymic temperament group as the cyclothymic make-up or constitution.

It is stated (Luxenburger and Schulz) that in the average population the percentage of definite manic-depressive psychosis is less than one-half of 1%, more exactly, 0.41%. If one adds the material of Luxenburger, Schulz, Brugger, Göppel, and Kattentidt, the figure is 0.15% in this segment of the population. This is probably altogether too small if we include the minor manic-depressive cases which never reach the institutions and which may pass unnoticed and are very commonly treated and studied as if they were neuroses. Certainly in private practice, the cases one classifies with manic-depressive psychoses constitute a considerable percentage of office work.

Rüdin is very frequently cited in the literature as an authority on the incidence of the inheritance of manic-depressive insanity, but we have failed to find that he has published any extensive and detailed statistical papers on the subject comparable with his schizophrenia studies, a fact also mentioned by Luxenburger. He (Rüdin) states that the incidence of the disease among the siblings of manic-depressive children of manic-depressive parents is 40 to 65%. While the absolute value of this figure may be open to the same objections as were raised in the case of schizophrenia, there is indication that the manifestation of this disease as a hereditary character is higher than that of schizophrenia on the whole. The character is generally considered to be dominant. However, it must be stated that the figure obtained lags behind the ones one would expect, and the term *irregular dominance* might fit the biological situation better. In a more recent paper, Rüdin concludes that the incidence of manic-depressive psychosis is 25 times as high among the siblings of manic-depressive patients as in the average population, although the data for this statement are not conspicuous or detailed.

A recent original study of the inheritance of this disease with an attempt to subject the figures to a statistical analysis is that of Hoffmann. This study is especially interesting because he takes into account the hyperthymic temperament. The material is small, only 159 cases being included. It is divided into two groups: First, children with one parent suffering from manic-depressive psychosis; 31.4% of these children showed definite depressions and elations;

39.5% showed a definite hypomanic or depressive temperament; 60% were normal but with some cycloid traits in their temperaments, which, however, remained within normal limits. The second group consists of a total of 35 cases. 7 of these are children of parents both of whom were suffering from manic-depressive psychosis. 3 (42.8%) of these had manic-depressive psychosis and the other 4 had cyclothymic (hypomanic or depressive) temperaments. The next sub-group of this material is made up of 12 cases who were children of one manic-depressive and one hypomanic parent. 5 (41.6%) of these children had manic-depressive psychosis, and there was a total of 7 out of 12 (50.8%) who had cyclothymic temperaments. If one adds to these, those cases with slight cyclothymia within normal limits, there were altogether 80.3% out of the total of 12 cases who may be called of the manic-depressive temperament or who had frank manic-depressive psychosis. The last sub-group of this material includes 16 cases who are children of one manic-depressive parent and one slightly hypomanic parent. 2 of these children were manic-depressives (12.5%); 5 were cyclothymic (31.2%), and adding to these the slightly cyclothymic within normal limits, there were 12 cases with positive involvement. 4 of the siblings were normal.

By plotting all these groups together, one finds the following figures for the descendants of one manic-depressive and one cyclothymic parent:

manic-depressives—10 out of 35 (28.5%)
cyclothymics in addition to the manic-depressives—19 out of 35 (54.6%)
adding slight cyclothymics within normal limits—22 out of 35 (62.8%)
normals—37.2%

Hoffmann discusses 31 more cases where one parent was manic-depressive, while the other is described as a schizoid personality. The distribution here was not fundamentally different from that cited above. Hoffmann also considers the question whether or not sex-linked factors may be acting in manic-depressive psychosis, but his groups are too small to be of any validity, and we may omit this factor in the consideration of the inheritance of manic-depressive psychosis.

The most recent German study on the subject is that of Luxenburger. He gives about the same figures as Rüdin and Hoffmann, namely, a probability for children of manic-depressive parents to develop the disease in 32%. However, the way that Luxenburger obtains these results is open to most serious objection. For the most part, he used Hoffmann's old material and merely rearranged it statistically. Altogether this material includes 162 children of manic-depressive parents, and there is no clear statement as to the number of families from which they come. We do not think that general conclusions are warranted from such a small group. They do not fit well with Banse's studies, to which Luxenburger himself refers, who found that in a family of altogether 2,473 members only 3.5% were definitely manic-depressive. Where practical eugenics is concerned, however, Luxenburger advises great caution and points to the fact that from marriages of manic-depressive couples children may emerge who do not have the genotype for manic-depressive insanity but only partial characters of it, which may be of great positive social and eugenic value. He emphasizes the principle of "Nicht Schaden!" (Don't do damage) and advises a strongly individual consideration in every case. Luxenburger himself points to the fact that manic-depressives, as a group, are socially productive and successful. He demonstrates clearly that in the families of manic-depressives, there are about four times as many members of the higher social strata than in the average population (23.3:8.7%). This fact he discovers from material of 1,502 members of manic-depressive families compared with 2,288 members of the average population.

We here abstract the paper on manic-depressive psychosis by Pollock, Malzberg, and Fuller:

We may test the applicability of the Mendelian theory to the inheritance of manic-depressive psychosis by an analysis of the siblings of the 155 probands admitted to the Utica State Hospital.

Of the original 155 family histories, it was necessary to eliminate 9 from the analysis owing to the incompleteness of the records. Of the remaining 146, there were 82 families in which both parents were outwardly normal, presumably producing matings of the DR x DR variety.

We may next consider separately a series of 48 families in which one parent might be classified as DR. In 26 of the families the other parent was described as nervous; in 14 as alcoholic, in 4 as psychopathic, and in 4 as suicidal. If we classify all of the latter as recessives, the matings would be of the DR x RR variety.

We may summarize our results in the statement that the observed frequency of mental disease among the siblings of patients with manic-depressive psychoses is inconsistent with a mode of inheritance based upon the supposed existence of Mendelian unit characters. We cannot reverse the argument, however, and conclude that because Mendelism is inapplicable, that inheritance therefore plays no part in the transmission of mental diseases. We have shown, on the contrary, that the frequency of mental disorders among the siblings, especially of manic-depressive psychoses, is significantly in excess of the total expected in populations selected at random. This was shown to be especially significant in connection with the siblings of female probands with manic-depressive psychoses. There appears to be, therefore, a familial basis for the development of mental disorders in many cases, although the underlying laws of their manner of transmission are not yet understood.

Other studies, such as that of Paskind, need only mention in this survey, since his data are computed from material studied on a polymorphous basis, which include alcoholism, apoplexy, senile dementia, psychopathic personality, and suicide as the hereditary taints.

An interesting question is the hereditary relationship of manic-depressive psychosis and dementia praecox. We may ask, is there a common factor in these two psychoses, which are the most important of the so-called endogenous psychoses? The frequency of dementia praecox among the siblings of manic-depressive patients is far less than among the siblings of general paresis and epilepsy and also considerably less than in the average population. The same is true concerning the incidence of manic-depressive psychosis among the siblings of schizophrenics.

We may summarize the situation in respect to manic-depressive psychosis as follows: Fewer cases than in schizophrenia have been studied and the statistical value of most of the publications is not high. It is safe to say that manic-depressive psychosis is inheritable; that whether in mild or severe form it manifests itself in a considerable number of the descendants or collaterals of those who have this disease. In its severe form it does not seem to be nearly so widespread as dementia praecox.

c. *Feeblemindedness*

The outstanding defect in all the discussion on feeblemindedness and its heredity has been the tendency to lump all the feebleminded together and to discuss feeblemindedness as if it were a unit. A preliminary consideration of the subject-matter shows that the case of feeblemindedness may be divided up into several main groups: (1) the cases due to sporadic cretinism; (2) Mongolian imbecility; (3) the organic brain diseases, that is, those in which the condition can fairly well be traced to brain injury at birth or infectious disease before or after birth; (4) the questionable so-called syphilitic feebleminded. (There is a considerable literature to show that this question cannot be said to be settled at the present time.) (5) Cases of microcephalus, cases of hydrocephalus in each case associated with feeblemindedness; (6) amaurotic idiocy; and (7) the mass of the feebleminded in whose cases no definite pathology has been established and which are only known as they manifest themselves by lower mentality. It is in this unclassified group that we find the feebleminded families, and it is concerning its relationship to this aggregation, which is probably not uniform in its composition, that the discussion concerning inheritance has mainly arisen.

Concerning *sporadic cretinism,* the literature as to heredity is meager, but none of the work indicates that heredity is an important factor. Hill states that he has seen three cases in which heredity factors were present, but apparently in these cases hyperthyroidism of some pathological type existed in the mother. In the rest of his series of 30 cases, there was no evidence of any hereditary influence at all. In Myerson's studies of the cretins at Wrentham and Waverley, heredity was definitely declared to be of no discernible importance.

Mongolism: The nature of Mongolism is at present unknown. It is probably related to some genetic disorder but usually occurs, as the whole literature attests, in normal families (even in one of twins) and bears no relationship to mental disease or feeblemindedness; that is to say, whatever its genetic constitution may be, and even this is doubtful, it is not the heredity of feeblemindedness or mental disease. Moreover, the Mongolians themselves do not marry and so far as is known are usually sterile. In one case reported (Dietrich and Berkley) a grown-up Mongolian idiot girl gave birth to a child that was not a Mongolian idiot.

Concerning *organic brain diseases,* there are two main points of view: first, that while trauma and an encephalitis produce mental deficiency, a constitution of an appropriate type is necessary for this result to be obtained. Thus, Jacobi and Konstantinu state that among cases that have undergone birth trauma three times as many result in feeblemindedness, if the parents were feebleminded than if the parents were normal. They state that this proves an endogenous factor even in the acquired forms of mental deficiency. Their argument is a little difficult to follow. The children who are born from feebleminded parents might well have been feebleminded if no trauma had occurred, whereas the probabilities are that the children of the normal parents would not have been feebleminded if the trauma had not occurred. On the whole, the literature may be stated as favoring the following points of view: if damage to a brain takes place early and in sufficient degree the best constitution for mental development may be thwarted and the result be feeblemindedness.

Concerning *microcephalus* and *hydrocephalus,* this may be stated—the former appears to be genetically determined, in that it occurs in family groups as a sporadic manifestation, but without any definite relationship to other deficiencies or the psychoses. Hydrocephalus is frequently environmental, following as it does meningitis or any pathological condition in which the communication between the ventricles and the subarachnoid space becomes closed off. However, it is also of congenital origin.

It is of interest to note that in the laboratory two distinct strains of mice exist which throw hydrocephalic individuals as Mendelian recessive characters.

Amaurotic idiocy occurs in families, in siblings as well as in collateral lines. But frequently an identical hereditary taint is absent. Of 12 cases of Gradle and Folk, identical hereditary taint could be established only in 3 cases. Consanguinity of the parents appears to favor the manifestation of the disease (Cordes and Horner). It occurs predominantly in Hebrews, but also in other racial groups (Gradle and Folk, Cordes and Horner). Amaurotic idiocy, however, is not primarily a mental disease but probably a symptom of a generalized disturbance of lipoid metabolism (Bielschowsky, Kufs).

The Subcultural Group

E. O. Lewis proposes the term "subcultural" for that group of mental defectives who represent the lower part of the frequency distribution curve of intelligence for the general population, separating them from another group which he terms the "pathological types" of mental defectives, that is, cases in which mental deficiency is associated with gross physical disease or deformity.

He gives an analysis of 100 families containing subcultural mental defectives selected on the basis of having at least one child certified as mentally defective and who appears to be of pure subcultural type. The families consist of parents and their immediate offspring only. The average I.Q. of the defectives (the propositi) through whom the selection was made was 50. Their families were all investigated personally and the available members were classed as follows:

Superior intelligence	125
Normal	100
Dull	75
Mentally defective	50

It was not possible, he stated, to measure by standard tests, but by school reports, histories, etc. Some of the causes for variability in intelligence are to be looked for in hereditary factors, but the gradation of intelligence in different individuals is steady and continuous and, he states, we cannot hope to find a single Mendelian character determining these variations.

The author tested data from 100 families against the hypothesis that a single gene determines the variation in intelligence from one individual to another, and he came to the conclusion finally that his figures agreed nearly enough with the expected ratio to warrant the assumption of the likelihood of multifactorial inheritance. He states also that there are quite definite indications that environment does play a part in the variations of intelligence, even in the subcultural group and believes that children born to the mother after the age of 35 are more likely to be low in intelligence than those born to younger mothers.

Thus, an important question arises—whether or not there is a truly qualitative difference between feeblemindedness and normal mentality. It is obvious that normal mentality runs a range from the low grade individual, capable of getting through grammar school and of carrying on an occupation which involves mainly the use of his muscles and, to a certain extent, the use of his mind, who makes his social adjustments and cultural acquisitions on this plane, to the genius whose mind encompasses the abstract relationships of man in the universe and whose work and formulations guide the destinies of his fellow-men. Between the low grade individual and the genius is what seems, at least on cursory examination of mankind, to be a series of powers and abilities which pass almost insensibly from low gradeness to mediocrity to high grade ability into talent and genius. This may not be the case, and there may be actual qualitative hereditary factors which operate, but the question has not yet been settled, and the relationship of mental ability and cultural environment is so intimate that no formulation can safely be made except to state that ability, in large measure, is innate, springs up sporadically in the most unlikely places and disappears where it might be expected, but requires in all instances an environment which is favorable for its manifestation.

Between the low grade individuals who form the lower bracket of so-called normality and the high grade feebleminded seems to be only a step, and that this step can be bridged by intensive effort and culture, favorable social environment seems to be definitely established by the work of Freeman, Holzinger and Mitchell, which we shall discuss later.

The literature on the inheritance of feeblemindedness may be divided up into several groups, some of which we need only mention and others which we will consider at length. There is, first of all, the genealogical studies of the royal families of the feebleminded—the Nams, Jukes, the Kallikaks, the Tribes of Ishmael, the Hill-Folk, etc. From the publications on these families, one would believe that they are representative of feeblemindedness in general; that these people are immensely prolific; and that heredity in these cases has been clearly established. Much of the sensational literature on this subject seems motivated by the desire, laudable enough, to save the race from being swamped by the low grade and the feebleminded.

The objections to including this type of research under the caption of science and to giving it serious consideration have been pointed out by Myerson. In the first place, these families, if they are feebleminded, are not representative of the mass of the feebleminded. As has been stated previously, Popenoe and Brugger, working in different communities, found that the mass of the feebleminded in the institutions come from the lower middle class of the population and are representative of the community as a whole, with the exception of the highest grade groups financially and socially. In the second place, the technique of investigation is open to serious and destructive criticism. The work has largely been done by field workers who have passed judgment rather too glibly and surely on people dead three, four or five generations, concerning whom no real authentic information could be obtained. For example, these workers have *known* that someone dead for a generation or two was syphilitic; they have made the diagnosis of moron by inspection and by the briefest of views, and they, therefore, made too light of very difficult problems and have been certain where only uncertainty exists. In all these instances, the individuals, although they probably contain a larger quota of feebleminded than the total population, have represented groups more or less sequestered who have lived in milieus of low cultural planes and have been subjected to a tradition and environment of a malign type.

Studies of the families of the feebleminded in Massachusetts have not revealed the Nam or Kallikak type of families. On the contrary, it has shown that there are always good collateral branches and that the totality of social damage inflicted on society has not been nearly so considerable as indicated.

A second type of research is one which is based on the polymorphic idea entirely and in which alcoholism, hemiplegia, senile dementia, syphilis, criminality, peculiar personality and vagrancy, to say nothing of Bright's disease, blindness, deformity, etc., have been set up as etiologic and hereditary factors bearing upon the feeblemindedness of the propositus.

In the face of Diem's work on the heredity of the normal and of Elderton's and Pearson's work on the descendants of the alcoholic, in which it is shown that these descendants are certainly not inferior to the descendants of abstainers, in view of all the doubts cast upon such an extensive amplification of a unit character of psychopathic inheritance, we may exclude such studies, even though, as in the case of the work done by Davenport and his associates, the formulation has finally been Mendelian and the point of view ostensibly scientific.

An example of the type of work done which is based too rigidly, it seems to us, on a theory is the paper by Rosanoff in which he states that mental deficiency seems to be consistently more common in the male than in the female sex. This is most strikingly shown in opposite-sex twins. Among 27 pairs of this kind, both had mental deficiency in 11 instances, the male alone in 11 instances, and the female alone in 5 instances. It appears in a consistent way that girls make a slightly better showing than boys in intelligence tests and in scholastic records. Rosanoff concludes that any relative excess of mental deficiency in the male sex must be attributed to a sex-linked factor.

In the criticism of the above, it may be stated that the

number of cases is altogether too small for any such conclusions, and no statistical device can overcome this deficiency. In one large hospital one of the committee found many more cases of female families than of male, and in a neighboring hospital, the reverse was discovered. Moreover, to state that the female is biologically more intelligent than the male on the basis of a few points of superiority in the intelligence test scores is to fly in the face of the historical fact that the intellectual and artistic accomplishment of the race, up to the present time, is masculine.

Some Researches of Large Scope

The British Commission on Sterilization gives the results of an English inquiry as to the descendants of mental defectives. The total number of cases reported on was 3,733, the mother being defective in 3,247 cases and the father in 486. The sex discrimination is explained by the statement that the defective mother is more likely to be brought to the notice of the local authorities than the defective father. This is especially the case if the children are illegitimate or neglected.

These defectives produced 8,841 children of whom 2,001 or 22.5% have already died. The percentage of deaths is striking and this confirms the conclusion drawn from other evidence furnished to us that the mortality among defectives and the offspring of defective stocks is abnormally high. This high rate is doubtless due in some measure to the poor environment in which many defectives live and to their inability to take proper care of their children. But the mortality appears to us too great to be attributable entirely to bad environment and parental inefficiency, and in our view it goes far to confirm the evidence from other sources of a relation between mental defect and inherent poor physique.

In the analysis of the figures, children under seven have been excluded, because mental defect in very young children, except of the lowest grade, cannot be ascertained with any certainty. The significant groups are those between seven and thirteen, and those over thirteen. The most striking point which emerges from a comparison of these two groups is, that in the latter group, the percentage recognized as definitely defective as compared with the retarded shows a marked increase and the percentage classified as superior shows a decrease . . .

Excluding the cases classified as 'unascertained,' that is, about whom no definite information was available, there were 1,802 children between seven and thirteen of whom 305 or 16.9% were classified as defective and 423 or 23.5% as retarded. Only 21 or 1.2% were superior. In the second group, children over thirteen, out of a total of 1,848, the number of defectives was 599, or 32.4%, and of retarded 240 or 13%. Only 10 or .5% were superior. The higher proportion of defectives as compared with retarded children in this group suggests that many of the children in the group seven to thirteen who were classed as retarded will later be found to be defective. Taking the two classes together we find that in the first group 40.4% of the children still living were mentally subnormal, and in the over thirteen group the percentage had risen to 45.4.

An important statement is made by the British Commission that the groups of cases in which morbid heredity and environmental conditions are both present is a much larger one. The percentage of cases coming within this class is estimated differently by different observers; according to the Colchester inquiry it amounts to 62%. The Commission, however, definitely states that there is no direct association between slums and mental deficiency, although it may well be that where hereditary predisposition is present, slum conditions act as a contributory factor in accentuating the results of this predisposition; "but we have been unable to find any evidence that slum conditions, though plainly disadvantageous in a general way to physical and mental health, are in themselves responsible for causing mental deficiency."

The results of this inquiry are summed up thus:

1. In many cases of mental defect there exists in the family some form of mental abnormality, that is, insanity, psychoneurosis, epilepsy, defect or dullness. In the majority of such cases

there is evidence of heredity but the mode of transmission is at present unknown.

2. In the case of certain rare forms of defect, not only is the fact of hereditary transmission known, but the method of transmission has been demonstrated.

3. It is probable that some mental defect is determined by a combination of genetic and environmental factors.

4. Some mental defect is not inherited, that is, the defect is acquired after conception as a result of environmental causes. There is no evidence that such defect is transmissible to subsequent generations.

5. Low grade mental defect is more frequently associated than is high grade defect with environmental factors, and it appears to be fairly equally distributed among all classes of society.

6. There is some evidence that conditions operating during the intra-uterine period may produce mental defect, but very little is at present known on this point.

7. High grade mental defect occurs proportionately more frequently in the lowest social stratum than in the rest of the population. In this stratum there appears to be an unduly high incidence of mental defect, insanity, intellectual dullness, epilepsy, as well as tuberculosis and other physical defects. Cause and effect of the conditions found in the social problem group are debatable, but it is possible that selective mating may to a large extent account for this concentration of physical defects and mental defects and disorders. There is evidence that in the poorest districts neighbor marries neighbor, and like marries like.

8. There is no evidence that parental alcoholism is responsible for any appreciable amount of mental defect. Recent research on this matter casts doubt on some of the earlier conclusions based on animal experiments.

9. Our evidence does not indicate any causal connection between tuberculosis and mental defect.

10. Syphilis is responsible for some, though an undetermined amount of, mental defect.

11. It is impossible in the present state of our knowledge about the causation of mental defect to forecast with certainty whether a child of any given union will exhibit mental abnormalities. It can, however, be shown that, whether the cause be bad heredity or adverse environmental conditions, or both, the children of parents one or both of whom are mentally defective are, on the average, below the normal, and our inquiry shows that nearly

one-third of such children as survive are likely to be defective, and more than two-fifths must be expected to exhibit some degree of mental abnormality.

Two American researches may be cited at this point as representing two types of material found, first, in the community, and second, in an institution. The importance of these two researches is that they were carried out in the same general community, that is, in Massachusetts, where there have for a long time existed good hospitals for mental deficiency and where at the same time community inquiry and community interest has been high.

Neil A. Dayton studied 3,553 children who are classified by him as the group who do poorly in school but who are not yet committed and, in the main, will not be committed; in other words, individuals who may be classified as mentally defective in the upper group and who represent undoubtedly a larger cross-section of the mentally defective population than ever is represented in the institutions:

1. Heredity, as recorded in the 3,553 school clinic examinations, reveals that feeblemindedness is present in one or both parents in approximately 7% of the cases, mental disease in approximately 3% of the cases, and epilepsy in 1% of the cases. The comparison in heredity made with cases in the Wrentham State School, seems to indicate that the inheritance of mental defect is more obvious in institution cases than in school clinic cases.

2. Approximately 72% of the children examined were feebleminded.

3. Sixty per cent of the children examined were unsuccessful in their attempts to pass the first grade in school.

4. There is little difference in the order of birth of these retarded children and children in the general population.

5. Physical defects were very common. In fact, there were but 26 children out of the total of 3,553 who were without physical defect. Four children out of five had defective teeth or tonsils. One retarded child out of four had defective vision or hearing, one out of six had a defective heart or defective circulation. One

out of seven had a nervous disease or disorder. One out of seven had a disorder of the bones.

6. Height and weight revealed but little variation from accepted averages in the general child population.

7. Four hundred and fifty-eight cases having two examinations at a mean interval of one and one-half years, show an increase in the mean mental age from seven years to eight years. During this period, the mean intelligence quotient decreased from .76 to .73. There were intelligence quotients which increased, but there were more showing a tendency to decrease, and consequently the mean of the second examination was depressed three points. Whether this decrease is significant or not is not yet settled, because of insufficient numbers.

It is unfortunate that in this study no personal examination was made of the siblings, since this would have thrown considerable light upon the relationship between the various mental diseases in the parents as well as their normality to the amount of feeblemindedness produced in the descendant generation. However, insofar as it goes, it very definitely indicates that the parents of the feebleminded are more often feebleminded than would be expected by random sampling. Secondly, that mental disease is not especially prominent since the amount of mental disease in the average population is to be rated as certainly near 3%. Epilepsy does not appear conspicuously insofar as these figures go. They are against polymorphism. They do not indicate a Mendelian heredity, but they do definitely show that a hereditary factor is at work.

The graph on page 124 taken from Dayton indicates clearly the difference between institutional and non-institutional cases as exemplified in the studies made by him and those made by Myerson and his associates.

It is to be also emphasized that physical defects are very common. It can hardly be stated that these had a benign result on the mentality of the children. It can hardly be claimed on the basis of our present understanding that they definitely caused the feeblemindedness or the retarded condition. Nevertheless, improvement in the general mental status of the children could be expected in some measure by the elimination of these defects.

The second study to which we have reference is the one to which Dayton alludes, the study of the Wrentham State

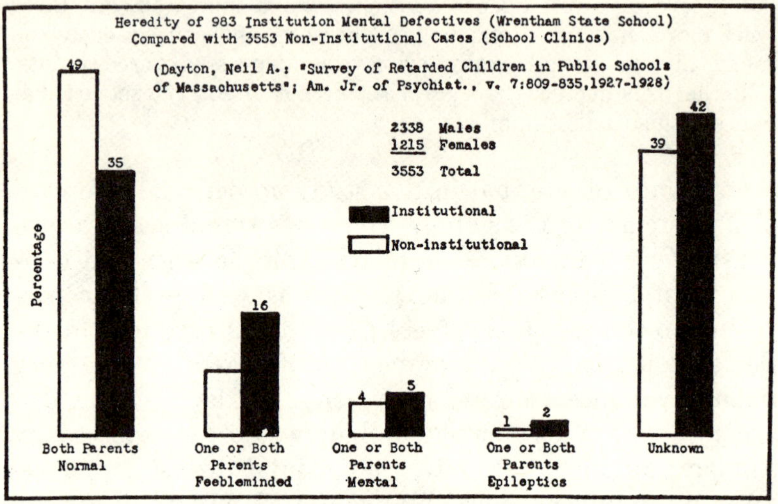

School, undertaken by Myerson and his associates and carried on for several years. This study has several defects. First, that although the author has throughout insisted that feeblemindedness should not be considered as a unit, he does consider it as such in taking the admissions in a consecutive way to the Wrentham State School. Thus, this group would include cretins, Mongolians, cases of organic brain disease, microcephalics, hydrocephalics, as well as the unclassified group. However, the ratio of these cases is small and does not to any important degree depreciate the result. The fundamental criticism of this and other types of work is that the siblings and parents were not personally studied. (See following table.)

Table IX —*Number of Families of Patients admitted for the first time to Wrentham State School having specified Number of Siblings (including Patient) with Percentage of Feeble-minded Children among them — 1920–1925, inclusive, with the expected percentages if Feeble-mindedness Behaves as a Simple Recessive* *

Families Having Specified Number of Siblings (Including Patient)

	Total Families	1		2		3		4		5		6		7		8		9		10+	
		Number	Per cent of Feeble-minded	Number	Per cent of Feeble-minded	Number	Per cent of Feeble-minded	Number	Per cent of Feeble-minded	Number	Per cent of Feeble-minded	Number	Per cent of Feeble-minded	Number	Per cent of Feeble-minded	Number	Per cent of Feeble-minded	Number	Per cent of Feeble-minded	Number	Per cent of Feeble-minded
Observed	591*	76	100.	97	60.	115	47.	115	37.	82	30.	25	23.	5	30.	25	23.	12	14.	39	16.
Expected	– †	–	100	–	57 ± 2	–	43 ± 2	–	37 ± 2	–	33 ± 2	–	30 ± 3	–	29 ± 6	–	28 ± 3	–	27 ± 4	–	26 ± 1

*591 out of 983 admissions (about 60 per cent) had information as to size of family and number of feeble-minded siblings. We have here discarded "unknowns" on the assumption that, were the information known instead of unknown, the meaning of the table would not be materially changed. We have assumed that the probability of obtaining information as to the number of feeble-minded siblings is not correlated with the size of the family; also that where the number of feeble-minded siblings is known and nothing is stated about the children who are not declared feeble-minded, they are not feeble-minded. In addition patients have been counted as representing separate families; that is, a family has been counted twice, or in rare instances three times. It is not uncommon in schools for the feeble-minded to have a number of related siblings under care. This particular circumstance lessens somewhat the statistical significance one would attach to the above percentages.

The observed distribution includes both the classified and the unclassified. When the unclassified cases were analyzed by themselves, the same observed ratios were noted as were found for the group as a whole. Whatever differences occur were found to be not significant statistically.

† The expected percentages in Table XVIII were estimated as follows: Let p = the chance of a feeble-minded person among siblings in the family, n = number of siblings in a family, N = number of families. In the general population then by chance alone we should expect the siblings of the family to be distributed according to the terms of the expansion of $(p+q)^n$. But the above data was selected obviously so that it contained no families in which no siblings were feeble-minded. Therefore $\Sigma(p+q)^n$ in the selected sample is $1-q^n$ instead of unity. The mean of the sample is therefore $\frac{np}{1-q^n}$ and the expected proportion of feeble-minded in the family of n siblings is $\frac{p}{1-q^n} = P$. The standard deviation of the above distribution is

$$\sigma = \sqrt{\frac{npq + n^2p^2}{1-q^n} - \frac{n^2p^2}{(1-p^n)^2}}$$

and the s. d. of the proportion P is

$$\sigma P = \sqrt{\frac{pq}{n(1-q^n)} + pP - P^2} = \sqrt{P\left(\frac{q}{n} + p - q\right)}$$

The mean proportion of N samples of n siblings is $\frac{\Sigma P}{N}$ and the s. d. of the mean $\frac{\Sigma P}{N}$ is $\frac{\sigma P}{\sqrt{N}}$.

Some estimate of the p must be made in order to evaluate these expressions. If we assume that feeble-mindedness is a character which behaves as a Mendelian recessive then we can let $p = \frac{1}{4}$. On this assumption the above expected proportions with their standard deviations have been computed. The agreement of the observed percentages with the expected percentages is very good except for the families of 9 and 10 siblings where the number of feeble-minded observed is significantly less than that which is theoretically expected.

* From Myerson and Elkind.

From this analysis the following conclusion was reached:

> Bearing in mind that throughout the analysis of the material it was generally assumed that a trait or factor was negative or did not exist if no observation was made as to that trait or factor, our study suggests the hypothesis that feeblemindedness of the unclassified type behaves as a simple recessive. The import of this conclusion is limited for the observations were of the institutionalized feebleminded and neglected the larger body of the feebleminded outside of institutions. The data show that social and economic factors play a large part in the admission of the feebleminded to training schools, and this fact further limits the significance of this hypothesis.

The study of Myerson and his associates also indicates that the amount of general inferiority is much greater in the feebleminded of the lowest level than those of the middle level, and these are inferior to the individuals at the highest level. It also appears from this study that convulsions are more common among the idiots than among morons and that in a general way this association may be related to the organic defectiveness of the idiot. A further conclusion appears from this study—the data from the Fernald School showed there was neither an excess nor a deficiency of mental disease among the parents while the data from the Wrentham School showed a significant excess of mental disease among the parents.

Wildenskov has published a monograph entitled, "Investigations into the Cause of Mental Deficiency." His general attitude is that there is a considerable percentage of exogenous feeblemindedness in the community, although the bulk of cases are probably on a hereditary basis. He does not attempt to formulate any definite hereditary mechanism operating in these cases. An interesting finding is here cited—that a lower moral and social standard, such as illegitimate birth, in the slightly mentally defective is almost four times more frequent than in the severely mentally defective and the parents of the slightly defective in comparison with the parents of the severely defective come three and a half times more often from the lowest social strata. It is the opinion of the committee that the number of cases (100) is too few for authentic conclusions.

An interesting and important angle of the problem of feeblemindedness is presented by Dayton, who made an extensive study of the influence of "size of family" upon the

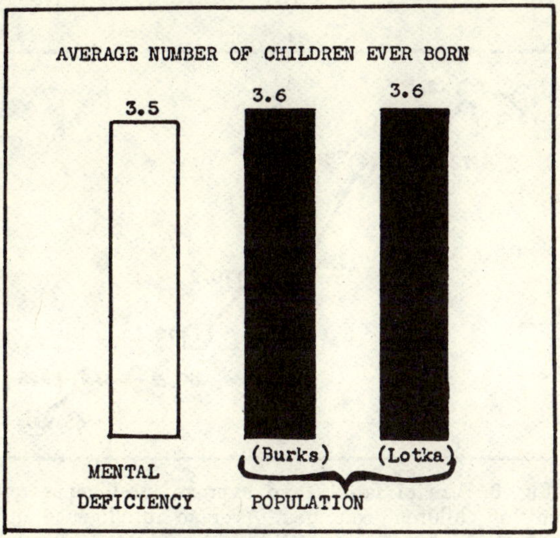

Fig. 5. Correct average number of children ever born: Families involving mental deficiency compared with the general population.[1]

[1] Dayton, Neil A.: Influence of size of family upon the characteristics of the mentally deficient. Am. J. of Psychiat., 91, 4, (Jan.) 1935, pp. 804, 805.

characteristics of the mentally deficient. The finding relevant to the present discussion is that with proper correction of the error of selection, the average number of children born in families of the feebleminded does not differ significantly from that of the general population. It is 3.5 per family as compared with 3.6 of the general population. (Fig. 5.)

This paper also considers the relationship between the size of the families from which the feebleminded come and the mental capacities and qualities of the siblings. *The average I.Q. of children born in families of different size decreases as the number of children increases.* The higher average I.Q. in the feebleminded group occurs in the children born in the smaller families, while the lower average occurs in the children from the larger families. A relatively higher average of 73.5 I.Q. occurs in the families of 2 children and a low average of 68.9 in the family groups of more

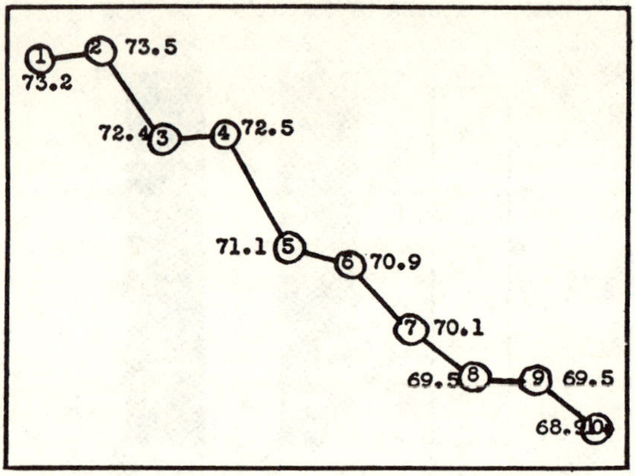

Fig. 6. Size of family and average intelligence quotient of children examined. Average intelligence quotient of children from families of one to ten plus sublings ever born. (From Dayton.)

than 10 children. These differences are not great but the size of the sample (20,473 families) adds statistical significance to comparatively small differences. The interpretation of this fact is, however, entirely problematic at the present time. (Fig. 6.)

The number of physical defects increases with the size of the families (Fig. 7). This is confirmatory of Dayton's previous paper and observations made by Myerson. Also the environment is classified as increasingly poor as the size of the family increases (Fig. 8).

Dayton concludes that about 85.9% of the parents of

mental defectives are not defectives themselves but merely carriers, on the basis of the general distribution of the character of feeblemindedness in the population. Very interesting is his calculation of the expectation of the incidence of feeblemindedness for the siblings of mentally defective

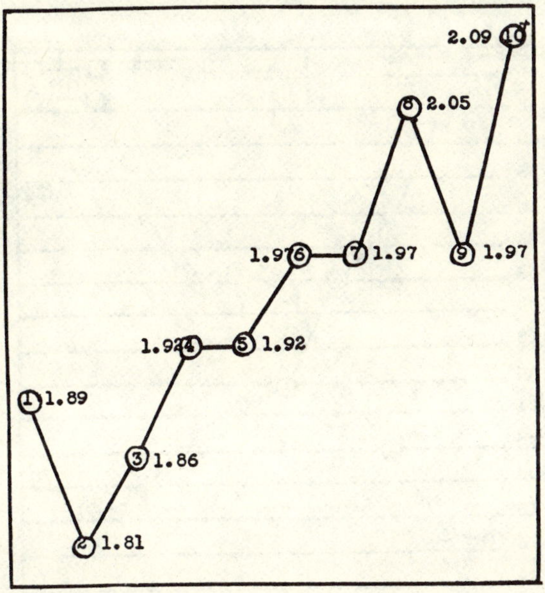

Fig. 7. Size of family and average number of physical defects per child examined. Average number of physical defects in families of one to ten plus siblings ever born.[1]

[1] Dayton, Neil A.: Influence of size of family upon the characteristics of the mentally deficient. Am. J. of Psychiat., 91, 4, (Jan.) 1935, pp. 814, 816.

children. There are 3 chances out of 40 that other children born in these families will be mentally defective; 5 chances that they will be retarded, and 32 chances that they will be average or normal.

There is a long and imposing literature on the subject of the inheritance of feeblemindedness, some of which we give in the references. In the main, the articles do not concern definite statistical studies made in large groups of cases, but this may be safely stated, that from whatever angle feeblemindedness is approached, if one excludes the cases where organic disease, cretinism, Mongolism, and other differentiated types of feeblemindedness are present, the results of the various studies show a larger proportion of inheritance of feeblemindedness than could be expected

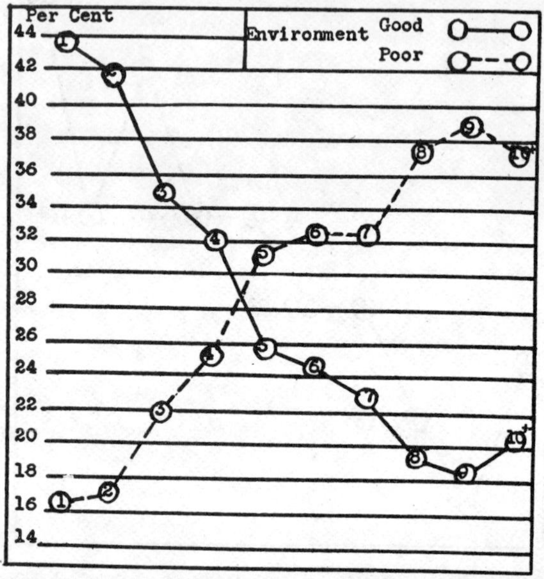

Fig. 8. Size of family and environmental status of homes of children examined. Environment in families of one to ten plus siblings ever born. (From Dayton.)

by any law of chance; in other words, that in a considerable segment of feeblemindedness, heredity plays a role of importance. It does not appear in the more careful studies made that mental disease and epilepsy are fundamentally related to feeblemindedness in a biologic sense. Furthermore, the literature, on the whole, is agreed that feeblemindedness, when hereditary, cannot be considered as a simple Mendelian recessive character; that if there is a

Mendelian inheritance, it is multifactorial which means, on the whole, that very little prediction can be made in a complete way as to the results of sterilization of the feebleminded themselves, nor could there possibly be, in the present state of our knowledge, any selection of individuals who themselves are not feebleminded to sterilize for the prevention of feeblemindedness.

Relationship of Intelligence and Environment

It seems to us important to discuss briefly the relationship of intelligence to environmental conditions as well as to heredity. Indeed, it is to be emphasized that the separation of heredity and environment is one of those dichotomies necessary to the human mind but essentially artificial in nature, and that in such a complex matter as the development of intelligence and ability, as well as in the establishment of moral character, the whole weight of the social heredity and immediate social environment must be of importance. At the same time, it must be stated that superior individuals are continually being born under conditions which we can only call at present inferior, so far as environment is concerned, and that inferior individuals appear upon the scene where the environmental conditions are favorable to the development of intelligence as we now understand it.

An interesting paper by Rosanoff and Inman-Kane, bearing on certain environmental factors in the genesis of low intelligence, is here cited:

> In the course of this work we have gathered records of 1,011 pairs of twins, (in which) either one or both twins of a pair have been afflicted with some mental disorder. In this material are included 234 pairs of twins with mental deficiency.
>
> The new material gathered especially for this study reveals that among 122 institutional cases of mental deficiency there were 26 or 21.31% in which there was premature birth (3 weeks

or more before term) or under-weight condition at birth (5½ lbs. or under), or both.

In a control group consisting of 9,782 births which occurred in five general hospitals in Los Angeles and Pasadena, the corresponding percentage was but 3.89. This figure is judged to be too high, as there was no way of making proper allowance for the abnormally high mortality of premature children during infancy and preschool age. It is estimated that the incidence of prematurity and of under-weight condition at birth among institutional cases of mental deficiency is no less than eight times as great as it is in the unselected population.

Our new material reveals further that among 146 children of elementary school age, who had been born prematurely or were in under-weight condition at birth, there were 15 cases (10.27%) of mental deficiency (I.Q. under 76), that is, relatively four times as many as the 2.63% found in Terman's series of 905 unselected children.[1]

This contrast, significant as it stands, is also probably an understatement of the case. Our follow-up investigations were conducted in the schools and therefore did not include the cases with the more severe results of head injury at birth, such as idiocy and the lower grades of imbecility, also those cases of mental deficiency which are complicated with the crippling effects of Little's disease or with epilepsy, all such cases being automatically precluded from school attendance.

The evidence seems conclusive to the effect that premature birth or under-weight condition at birth is an etiologic factor in mental deficiency. For the most part, if not entirely, the damage is caused by cerebral trauma occurring during birth. Premature and under-weight children are much more liable to suffer such damage at birth than are children born in full term and of normal weight. Prematurity and underweight condition at birth are much more common in multiple than in single births; for that reason, and probably by the same mechanism, mental deficiency is produced more often in twins than in single births.

Premature births or under-weight conditions at birth, or both per se, do not cause mental deficiency. In our group of cases no fewer than 19.29% of those in which the I.Q. had been ascer-

[1] It is of significance that early undernourishment particularly affects the brain and eyes. (See C. M. Jackson in: Jour. Exp. Zool., 19:99-156, 1915 and Anat. Rec., 61, suppl.: 28, 1935; quoted by T. Wingate Todd: "The Bodily Expression of Human Growth and Welfare"; Science, 82,212:181-186, Aug. 30, 1935.)

tained showed an I.Q. of over 115. The corresponding figure for Terman's group of 905 unselected children is but 11.55%.

Perhaps the most important study which has been done was carried out by the Chicago sociologists, Freeman, Holzinger, and Mitchell:

This study, made under the auspices of the University of Chicago, was a deliberate effort to discover whether the intelligence of the child is affected by the characters of the environment. They define intelligence very simply, as the quality of a person's behavior in dealing with intellectual problems. It is measured by the score which the individual makes upon adequate tests of intelligence. The tests used were the Stanford revision of the Binet-Simon Scale and the International Group Mental tests. Their idea was to compare persons who are alike in heredity, but who have been subjected to different environments, and, on the other hand, those who have diverse heredity, but have been under the influence of the same or of similar environment. The children tested were divided into groups, one a pre-test group who were children who had been given a Binet test before they were placed in their present homes. The authors summarize as follows:

The main problem of this investigation was the measurement of the effect of environment upon the intelligence of foster children. The detailed procedure by which this measurement was made has been described in the foregoing pages. This summary includes only a brief statement of the more important comparisons made and the conclusions which seem to be warranted.

1. A group of children were tested before placement and then retested after several years of residence in a foster home. A comparison of their ratings on the two tests gave evidence of a significant improvement in intelligence (as measured by intelligence test scores). A study of certain sub-groups showed that the children in the better foster homes gained considerably more than did those in the poorer homes. Furthermore, the children who were tested and adopted at an early age gained more than those adopted at a later age. These facts appear to indicate that an improvement in environment produces a gain in intelligence.

2. A comparison was made between the intelligence of siblings (brothers and sisters) who had been reared in different foster homes. The correlation between their intelligence was found to be lower than that usually found for siblings raised together.

The usual coefficient of fraternal resemblance is about .50, but it was found that for siblings separated before either of the pair was six years of age, the correlation was only .25. When the comparison was made for those whose foster homes were of different grade, the correlation was found to be only .19. These facts make it appear that a part of the resemblance between siblings reared together is due to the influence of a similar environment.

3. A group of siblings was divided into two groups by putting into one group the member of each pair who was in the better foster home and into the other group the one in the poorer home. The mean I.Q. of the group in the poorer homes was found to be 86, while that of those in the better homes was 95. An analysis of the conditions of adoption made it seem unilkely that there was any marked tendency for the brighter member of a pair of siblings to be taken into the better foster home. A random formation of two groups from pairs of siblings would give groups of equal intelligence. The superior intelligence of the siblings in the better homes appears, therefore, to give evidence that the character of the home affects the child's intelligence to a marked degree.

4. Two unrelated children reared in the same home were found to resemble one another in intelligence. The correlations between the intelligence of such unrelated pairs ranged from .25 to .37. This resemblance is probably due for the most part to the similarity of their environment.

5. The available information on the own parents of the foster children indicated that a large percentage were of defective mentality. If heredity were the only factor in the determination of intelligence, it would be expected that their children would be decidedly below the average. It was found, however, that their mean I.Q. was practically equal to the standard for children in general. Only 3.7% rated below 70, and these were those placed at relatively late ages. These facts seem to point quite clearly to the influence of environment upon intelligence.

6. In the case of 26 children studied, both parents were rated as feebleminded. If intelligence were inherited according to the Mendelian law, all of these children would be feebleminded. It was found, however, that only four had an I.Q. below 70 and these only slightly below. The average I.Q. of 81 for these 26 children is higher than would be expected according to the Mendelian law, but is considerably below that of the entire group of children studied. These facts appear to indicate that heredity

and environment are both influential factors in the development of intelligence.

7. The school progress of the children studied compares very favorably with that of the children in several large school systems.

8. In various groups comparisons were made between the intelligence of the children and the grade of foster home in which they had been reared. For the entire group of 401, the correlation between home rating and intelligence was found to be .48. The correlation between the intelligence of the children and the intelligence of their foster parents as measured by the Otis test was found to be .37. In the case of the children who had been tested before adoption, an initial correlation of .34 with home rating was raised to .52 after a period of residence in the foster home. These correlations would indicate that the character of the home is an important factor in the development of the child's intelligence.

9. The influence of the home is further shown by the fact that there is a correlation between early placement and intelligence and a slight relationship between the child's intelligence and the length of the time he has spent in the foster home.

10. A large percentage of the children studied had parents who were morally defective. In spite of this poor heredity, however, few cases of serious misbehavior were found among the foster children. It seems probable, therefore, that environment has been an important factor in determining their conduct.

11. In interpreting certain data of the study, it was necessary to know whether the apparent effect of good home environment could be accounted for by a selection of initially bright children by superior foster parents. The analysis of the data led to the conclusion that selection was not a large factor in the relationships. In the extreme cases in which the children were given a mental test before adoption, the correlation between this initial I.Q. and home rating was .34. In over eight per cent of the cases no test was made before adoption. Furthermore, a survey of the circumstances of adoption indicates that the intelligence of the child is not usually taken into account as a major consideration. Finally, for certain groups in which it would have been least possible to estimate the intelligence of the child, the correlation with home rating is as high as for other groups.

The enormously important significance of this paper is

substantiated by a German study, namely, "Effects of Predisposition and Environment Studied on Adopted Illegitimate Children." This paper studies the influence of heredity and environment from a material of adopted illegitimate children. The material has been gathered from the Youth offices (Jugendamt) of three large cities; 53 cases from Hamburg, 56 from Dresden, and 29 from Leipzig. The age of the adopted children at the time of adoption was under 2 years in 9.5%; 2 to 5 years in 44.5%, 6 to 10 years in 35%, and over 10 years in 11%. For the study of the influence of change of environment, the development before and after adoption was compared. The result was that before adoption, development was good in 42%; after adoption in 76%; mediocre before adoption in 38%; after adoption in 18%; bad before adoption in 20%; after adoption in 6%. (H. Reiter) . . . The study includes many other points, such as taint with tuberculosis, criminality, and analysis as to profession of natural and adopted parents.

We cite the above work to indicate that while heredity may operate to produce feeblemindedness, education and the improvement of the general milieu has its therapeutic place.

d. Epilepsy

This term has been dropped by many workers, who now speak of the convulsive disorders. The term epilepsy denotes an entity which no more exists than does "insanity." We retain its use in this report merely because the heredity studies in the literature bear this name.

In the case of epilepsy, it is necessary to state that we deal with a condition for which, in many cases, there are clear exogenous or environmental, exciting or precipitating causes. In this way, epilepsy differs definitely from manic-depressive psychosis and schizophrenia, in that for these latter conditions no such causes are clearly established. Moreover, animal experimentation has clearly shown that something very similar to epilepsy can be produced. This merely means that what is termed idiopathic epilepsy had better be classified as epilepsy of unknown origin.

The early workers on the heredity of epilepsy were quite unanimous as to the importance of heredity. Oppenheim himself states that a number of conditions are capable of producing epilepsy but apparently make their influence felt chiefly when the morbid predisposition is already present. But Oppenheim and, like him, Gowers were polymorphists and so they state that insanity in parents is the largest single hereditary factor, something not discovered by any of the later writers.

Thus, Spratling speaks of epilepsy as a disease dependent on nervous or degenerative disease in the parents more frequently than to any other cause. Binswanger, who is a firm believer in the polymorphic theory, gives as the main cause of epilepsy injury to the germplasm, citing these as the sources of the germplasm injury: chorea, the intoxications —alcohol, morphine, lead; the infections—tuberculosis, syphilis; constitutional diseases—anemia, leukemia, chlorotic disease, diabetes, gout, chronic hypertrophic arthritis—and finally, local diseases of the germ-forming organs, testicle and ovary through mechanical injuries, or degenerative or inflammatory processes.

It is easy to see that such a widespread net might also make normality a degenerative disease due to defect in the ancestors.

One of the most pretentious pieces of work is that done by Davenport and his group. Elsewhere one of us has criticized the work of Davenport, who came to the conclusion that epilepsy is a hereditary Mendelian character, although in later writings, he directly modified his opinion. What is called Mendelism in Davenport's work is merely polymorphism of the widest type. Thus, he has a legend which reads as follows: "Frequency of the different classes of mental conditions in the children of two mentally defective parents together with the mental condition of the grandparents, the parent's siblings (brothers and sisters), and other blood relatives about whom something is known." He then classifies the mental conditions by an alphabetical list which starts with A, alcoholic and ends with V, vagrant, and indicates many heterogeneous conditions which are exogenous as well as endogenous. Some of his characters represent a medley of causes, as for example, crippled, deaf, dwarf, eccentric, heart disease, etc.

Thom carried out a series of investigations bearing on the fate of the offspring of epileptics and cites, as a contrast, Echeverria's paper. With a similar number of married epileptics and a similar number of children, Echeverria found 273 epileptic offspring out of a total of 533, or over 51%, whereas Thom with siblings numbering 553 discovered only 10 epileptics. We cite Thom's conclusions in full:

1. The records of 1,536 epileptic patients admitted to the Monson State Hospital showed that 1 out of every 6 was married.
2. Eight per cent of the marriages resulted in children.
3. One hundred and thirty-eight marriages resulted in 553 offspring, an average of 4 to each marriage.
4. Of the 553 offspring it was possible to obtain a history of epilepsy in only 10 cases (1.8%).
5. Of these 10 epileptics, 6 died in infancy, 2 became confirmed epileptics, and 2 cases are arrested, one for seventeen years, the other for thirty-six years.
6. The study of the family history in 138 epileptics revealed epilepsy in one parent, 8 times, and the study of the offspring of these same patients showed that it had been transmitted 10 times; but in 2 instances there were 2 children in the same family who had convulsions, so that the epilepsy was inherited and transmitted in 5.8% of the cases.
7. These figures correspond more closely with the recent work of Stucklik, who found inheritance of epilepsy in epileptics direct from parent in 4.1% of 176 cases, than they do with the findings of Turner, Doran and Binswanger.
8. From the above it would appear that epilepsy is transmitted directly from parent to offspring less frequently than we have heretofore been led to believe.

Probably the two most important pieces of recent work are those by Brain in England and Calvert Stein in the United States. A summary of Brain's paper is as follows:

1. In a series of 200 epileptics a family history of the disease has been found in 28 per cent, as compared with a figure probably under 10 per cent in a control series from a hospital population.

2. A family history of the disease is obtained somewhat more frequently in the case of females than males.

3. The onset of the disease occurs in the first decade of life in a larger proportion of those with a family history of epilepsy than of those without such a history.

4. There was a history of early convulsions in the case of 28 per cent of 176 epileptics. Early convulsions were almost twice as common in epileptics with a family history of the disease as in those with none.

5. Epileptics have been found to transmit the disease to about 1 in 20 of their offspring, but considering the probable error of the small numbers, little stress can be laid on this proportion.

6. The proportion of first-born among epileptics is twice as high, and of second-born children half as high again, as in the section of the population from which the patients were drawn. It is suggested that the increased liability of first-born children to receive cerebral injury at birth is a factor likely to be responsible for the increased proportion of first-born among epileptics.

7. The incidence of insanity among the relatives of epileptics was found to be no higher than in the general population.

8. The facts are held to indicate that a predisposition, which in at least 28 per cent of cases is inherited, is an etiological factor in epilepsy.

9. Our present knowledge is not sufficient to render practicable the application of Mendelian principles to the inheritance of epilepsy.

Stein's method has been indicated in our previous discussion and we have criticized this method without intending, in any way, to disqualify the general results obtained by his study. First, as to the incidence of epilepsy itself or convulsive seizures in the immediate families of the patients and the similar incidence in the immediate families of the controls, the ratio is 18.1% as against 4.6% for the controls. Taking the total number of parents, siblings, and children, the occurrence of epilepsy is 3.7%, whereas in the controls numbering 4,684 parents, siblings and children, the percentage is 1.3. This is represented graphically by the following figure from Calvert Stein:

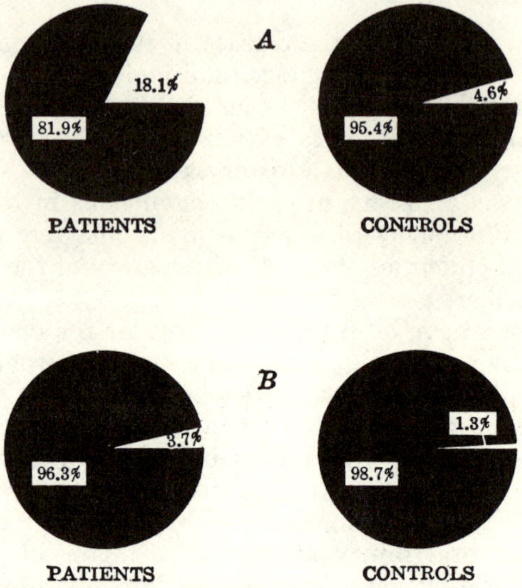

This figure expresses the relation between positive and negative histories for seizures in the immediate families of patients and controls. It presents what the committee considers to be the most important data in this study of heredity in epilepsy. The positive incidences of seizures (white) are here given their true proportions.

Thus, in A the positive incidence of seizures in the immediate families of 1,000 epileptics (18.1%) is nearly four times as great as that (4.6%) for the 722 controls. And in B—the percentage of the total number of 6,572 parents, siblings and children (3.7%) of the patients is nearly three times as great as (1.3%) in the 4,684 parents, siblings and children of the controls. But, on the other hand, in A—81.9% of the patients show no history of seizures in their immediate family and in B—96.3% of these 6,572 parents, siblings and children likewise show a negative history of seizures.

Stein points out, however, that the picture can be viewed from a different angle, that is, 81.9% of the patients give no history of seizures in their immediate families and 96.3% of the total number of relatives of the patients, parents, siblings, and children show a negative history of seizures. Looked at more directly, only 3.7% of the immediate relatives of the institutionalized epileptics themselves give a history of epilepsy.

The parental heredity of these patients is interesting, as contrasted with that of the normals. Stein states that seizures occur about eight times more frequently in the fathers of the patients (2.3%) than in the controls (0.3%); seven times more frequently in the mothers of the patients (3.5%) than in the controls (0.5%); and four times as often in the siblings of patients (12.4%) as in the siblings of the controls (3.1%), although the incidence of seizures in the total number of siblings is five times greater in patients (4.1%) than in the controls (0.8%). Seizures occur five times as often in the other relatives of the patients (14.2%) as in the other relatives of the controls (2.9%) and similar proportions exist for the remaining groups. Seizures occur more than four times as often in all or any relatives of the patients as in all or any controls.

We may ask at this point, what is the incidence of epilepsy in the community as a whole? We find very varying figures. Thus, Davenport puts the incidence of epilepsy at .5% among the drafted men of the United States Army in the World War, but obviously epileptics were excluded from the army, so that this does not represent the total population. Cobb believes the general incidence of epilepsy is one-third of 1%, so that, on the whole, the control figures of Stein seem warranted by the work of others, and the fact is definitely established that epilepsy is more frequent in the relatives of patients than in the general population.

However, it will be noted at once that there would be grave difficulties in detecting the parents who might give rise to epilepsy, for while 3.7% among Calvert Stein's material gave a positive history of epilepsy, 96.3% gave a negative history.

Our criticism of Stein's work on migraine has appeared before. He finds, on the whole, that it is a character which appears more frequently in the ancestors and collaterals of the epileptics than in the siblings and collaterals of the normals. We believe, however, that his figure is far too low for the normals.

He then takes up the question of the relationship of feeblemindedness and states that feeblemindedness occurs in much larger proportion in the families of the epileptics than among relatives of the controls. The incidence for the immediate family of the patients (17.0%) was nearly twice as high as for the controls (9.2%).

It is probable that certain forms of feeblemindedness bear at least some coincidental relationship to epilepsy. In Myerson's figures from the Walter E. Fernald School for the Feebleminded, it appears quite definitely that the lower type of feebleminded tend to have convulsions, while the higher type do not. This is also confirmed by Dayton's figures on the backward and feebleminded children of the community. Alcoholism appears four times as frequently in the parents of Stein's epileptics as in the parents of the non-epileptics, but it is pertinent to remark that it occurs many times more frequently than epilepsy itself does in the same parents. Consequently, if the figures are to be given credence, alcoholism is more important in the ancestry of the epileptics than epilepsy itself. Such figures do not take into account the frequency of alcoholism itself. Moreover, they need to be controlled by a study of the descendants of alcoholics as a separate research.

As we have stated before, Elderton and Pearson's figures definitely indicate that the descendants of the alcoholics do not suffer more from mental disease, epilepsy, and feeblemindedness than do the children of non-alcoholics. Moreover, it may be stated that one of the conspicuous races, or ethnic groups, the Jew, is on the whole a non-alcoholic people, yet no one has accused them of contributing less than their share of mental disease and epilepsy. What stands out as important from the work of Stein are his conclusions:

1. The results of this study do not justify the conclusion that the symptom-complex known as epilepsy, either *per se* or as migraine, or as any other neuropsychiatric disorder, is an inherited condition.

2. However, the higher incidence of neuropsychiatric disorders in the families of epileptics may well be explained on the basis of an existing potential or latent germplasm defect. It is likely that this defect or vulnerability furnishes more than usually fertile ground for the production of epilepsy by such known contributing factors as trauma, infection, birth injury, alcoholism, etc. In other words, it may be that this potential or latent germplasm defect, whatever it may be, requires a less severe blow than usual from the above named contributory or exciting factors, in order to activate it into the clinical condition known as epilepsy.

3. It is difficult to escape the conclusion that this germplasm defect or vulnerability appears in too large a proportion in the family histories of the patients, when compared with those of the controls, to be entirely accidental.

While we may in some measure accept these conclusions of Stein, there would be more merit to them if the controls had been selected from the same social group as the epileptics and the family histories obtained in the same way. However, allowing for these circumstances, the committee accepts the statement that epilepsy occurs more frequently in the descendants of the epileptics than in the descendants of the non-epileptics, and also agrees that the vast bulk of epileptics arise from families having a low incidence of epilepsy and who, in the main, are indistinguishable from the mass of the population.

This bears, of course, on the question of the prevention

of epilepsy by sterilization. The proportion of epilepsy in families makes it clear that if there is a Mendelian factor involved that no single unit recessive Mendelian character can be invoked as explaining its incidence. The proportions found are far too small. On any Mendelian basis, multifactorial characters have to be created. The difficulty with predisposition is that it is too vague a concept and has little practical validity. It is probable that the best efforts of science at the present time, insofar as the epilepsy problem is concerned, will be expended in the study of the pathology, chemistry, and general physical constitution of the individual patient himself in the hope of discovering both a pathogenesis and a cure.[1]

[1] It is interesting to note that at the last International Neurological Congress there was an important section on the epilepsies and not a single paper on heredity. In fact, one author, Jean Abadie, went so far as to state as follows: Epilepsy is not a neurosis; it is due to organic injury of the nervous centers. Epilepsy is not a hereditary disease; it is an acquired affection. The ancient doctrine of the so-called idiopathic epilepsy, that is, to be opposed to the symptomatic epilepsies should be completely abandoned.

Lennox in his important paper read at this Congress concluded:

"Abnormal states of body physiology in the form of alkalosis, of generalized cerebral anaemia or of anoxaemia are not a cause of seizures in the usual person with epilepsy. These states may, however, alter seizure threshold and precipitate seizures in persons subject to frequent petit mal.

"Petit mal seizures are associated with alterations in the electrical activity of the brain—very large, slow fluctuations in potential replacing the usual short, fast fluctuations. Alkalosis, anoxaemia and anaemia produce a similar change in electrical activity and perhaps act by integrating with and discharging the patient's neurological seizure mechanism."

He did not mention either constitution or heredity, and similarly with the other papers at the Congress.

It seems to be a general rule that where little is known of a disease, the more is ascribed to heredity; where more is known, less is ascribed. The paradigm of tuberculosis arises at once. In the early days of the nineteenth century, shrewd clinical observers ascribed the disease to heredity on much the same basis that we now ascribe the mental diseases to this factor, namely, that it occurs in family groups beyond the normal expectation. When the tubercle bacillus was discovered, the idea of heredity as the cause of tuberculosis disappeared, and then there surged to the front the concept of constitution, but as we have stated before, constitution may be hereditary, but it also may be acquired.

VII

CHRONIC PROGRESSIVE NEUROLOGICAL DISEASES

1. Chronic Progressive Chorea (*Huntington's Disease*). It is generally accepted that Huntington's chorea is a dominant, probably monohybrid character. About 50% of the offspring are likely to inherit the disease. Stone recently published an interesting paper on this subject, in which the history of our knowledge of the disease is given. The first description was that by W. Lyons in 1863 of four generations in one family. Huntington's description in 1872 brought out the main points, (1) its hereditary nature; (2) its association with mental symptoms such as the tendency to mental alteration and suicide; (3) appearance in adult life, and the fact that it never skips a generation to manifest itself in another.

There has been an attempt by Davenport also to link up this disease with others in a polymorphous fashion by studying 3,000 relatives of 962 propositi. He found among these relatives epilepsy in 39 cases, infantile convulsions in 19 cases; meningitis in 51 cases, hydrocephalus in 41 cases, feeblemindedness in 71 cases, and tic in 9 cases. To us, however, this reprcsents a not unusual or significant distribution of those diseases in a population.

It is generally agreed that males and females are equally affected, and that transmission occurs both through males and females (Worster-Drought and Allen; and Chapman). It has been stated that the disease never affects Hebrews. Worster-Drought and Allen suggest a lessened tendency to the disease in successive generations. This may probably be due to the fact that the character as a dominant one is being bred out. They also note a lessened expectation of life in those afflicted in successive generations. In the successive generations deafness and dumbness in childhood crop out here and there and also what may be called psychoneurotic states.[1]

2. Acute Forms of Chorea. There has also been a hereditary element suggested for the manifestation of rheumatic chorea and for a group of cases which may be described as acute and congenital chorea, but the observations are still too rare to be definitely conclusive.

3. Athetosis. Familial occurrence of hereditary degenerative athetosis was first described by Oppenheim and Vogt in a case of mother and daughter, both of whom presented an almost identical clinical picture. The daughter's brain was studied anatomically and she was found to have been suffering from a dysgenesis of the basal ganglia (status dysmyelinisatus). The association of this disease with myoclonus epilepsy has been recently observed by van Bogaert.

4. Friedreich's Ataxia. Friedreich's ataxia is a highly heritable disease. Both direct and collateral inheritance occurs, direct inheritance not being the rule and its rate of affliction being the highest among siblings. It has, however, been described in three successive generations—in the grandfather, mother, and son, by Naffziger and Shepardson, and in mother and two sons by Gordon. There are indications that the number of diseased individuals in a family increases with each generation (Giddings). A number of authors agree that the series of cases in every given family become afflicted with definite constancy at about the same age (Giddings).

[1] While the laboratory does not produce completely analagous cases of chorea, it is of some relevance that by inbreeding it is possible to produce two strains of mice, known as shakers, which are pure bred recessives.

The data seem to indicate that in this disease an atypically recessive character of rather high "penetrance" may be responsible. The curvature of the spine which is frequently found in this disease is considered to be secondary to the muscular weakness.

5. *Spastic Spinal Paralysis.* In this disease familial occurrence has been frequently described, especially among siblings, but also in direct and collateral lines. Especially interesting is the case of Schaffer concerning two brothers, with an anatomic study.

6. *Progressive Muscular Atrophy.* This disease occurs in families in direct line, vertically as well as horizontally, and in collateral lines. Cavanaugh and Tucker conclude that males and females are equally affected and probably transmit the disease equally.

Gordon describes the incidence of the disease (Charcot Marie Tooth type) in a man, 46 years of age, and in the cousin of his mother, both of whom had normal direct offspring. Worster-Drought described the same disease in mother and two children, both of them boys. Gordon thinks that the disease in general is transmitted by affected females to their male and female descendants. But we believe that the material available is not yet large enough to warrant this conclusion. There are, however, a great number of casuistic studies in the literature which it would be worth-while to plot together and to work up statistically.

7. *Muscular Dystrophy.* There is, in general, a similar type of inheritance as in the aforementioned groups in this disease. Cases are described in direct (vertical and horizontal) and in collateral lines (Monrad-Krohn, Rollin). Monrad-Krohn described the disease in two brothers, whose father presented rudimentary myopathic affection of one limb only.

8. *Myotonia (Thomsen's Disease).* This rather rare disease has been recorded as occasionally occurring familially.

It has been described in direct horizontal line (in brothers) by Elkington and Gunnar Böe. Barker recorded it in a brother, a sister, and one cousin on the father's side in one family. It has been stated that there was intermarriage in this family. Urechia, Retezeanu, and Dragomir recorded a similar disease (*paramyotonia*) in the collateral line in four generations in one family.

Other authors (Burke, Valdes Dias) fail to demonstrate evidence of hereditary transmission in their cases. Although there is some indication of inheritance in this disease, we do not believe that the evidence is conclusive enough as to deny any possibility of another, especially endocrine, etiology as Ruhemann did. In the case of Ruhemann the patient had sustained injury on the head, fracture of the nasal bone, fracture of the ribs, and injury of the testes. Two years later a myotonia developed. Ruhemann denies any connection of the accident with the disease on the basis that this disease is hereditary, in spite of the fact that no heredity has actually been demonstrated in this case. The data of Gunnar Böe, who found in two brothers who were suffering from the disease segmental spinal changes in the inferior dorsal cord, points to the fact that the disease may be due to alterations of the autonomic system of the spinal cord.

9. Syringomyelia. There are some cases reported of collateral and direct heredity in syringomyelia. Tenner reported it in father and daughter, van Bogaert in two sisters. Ostertag found it in a strain of inbred rabbits.

10. Infantile Diplegia and Monoplegia. There is some information that this disease may occur in siblings (Denzer, Baumann), but here other factors, such as intrauterine environment, are more likely to be operating.

11. Paroxysmal Paralysis. This rare disease has been described in two brothers and their father by Safran. The other cases recorded are not familial. Strauss thinks that there is some relation of the disease to carbohydrate metabolism, since in his case attacks were elicited by a high intake of carbohydrates.

12. Hereditary Optic Atrophy (Leber's Disease). Merritt and Kuhn have furnished data to indicate that a recessive character may be operating in this disease. There is also some possibility that the disease may be mainly transmitted by normal females to males, since usually only males are afflicted. In Kuhn's case two sons and two brothers of one woman were afflicted by the disease. Ferguson and Critchley, however, found the disease in females, namely, among siblings, consisting of one brother and three sisters. One of these sisters had also an ataxia of Friedreich's type in addition to the optic atrophy.

13. Diseases of the Peripheral Nerves. The familial occurrence in direct, horizontal, and vertical, and in collateral lines of Recklinghausen's neurofibromatosis has been reported frequently. Also the familial occurrence of nerve tumors, especially that of neurinoma of the eighth nerve, has been reported in direct line (mother and child).

VIII

CRIME

THE laws which invoke sterilization in relationship to crime are mainly directed against those guilty of such sexual offenses as rape and the so-called sexual perversions. Since people do not ordinarily rape and commit sexual perversions with the idea of procreation, and since procreation is extremely rare as a result of such offenses, castration would appear to be mainly a punishment and sterilization of no particular value, since it does not interfere with the sexual impulse. There is almost no evidence to show that criminality as such could be reached by sterilization, although there may be and there probably is a type of individual predisposed to crime by his constitution. What almost all the authors who have given the matter serious thought stress is the interplay between the environment and the individual as creating crime. Moreover, any definition of crime is social and that definition varies from place to place and from time to time. The term criminal, or criminalistic, is by no means unitary, therefore, and in reality crime is committed by people of varying types of mentality, personality and genetic constitution.

Perhaps the most important recent work showing a genetic constitution for crime was that by Lange in his now famous book "Verbrechen als Schicksal," in which he showed that certain identical twins committed crimes of similar type. This, however, proves very little, since there is still the interrelationship between the constitution of these identical twins and their environment to take into account. Later on, Lange himself in his article, "Verbrechen und Vererbung," points out the difficulty of recognizing the criminogenetic constitution. He states that eugenics must be modest. As a matter of fact, his identical twins who committed murder belong either to the affectless type of the schizophrenic or to the definitely hereditary feebleminded groups.

Mayer considers the "born" criminal as extraordinarily rare and states there may be one among 10,000 people, and even Rüdin points out that there may be an inheritance of a readiness to certain criminal social reactions which in favorable environmental conditions will not be elicited.

Heimberger who studied prison colonies in South Wales in Australia found that the progeny of a large number of the criminals who were sent there did not prove inferior, and Mayer refers to the work of Sticker, who states that the colony of criminals founded in 1728 in Botany Bay in South Wales has not become the source of criminalistic descendants.[1]

W. N. East made a medical investigation of the Boys' Prison in Wandsworth and found that in a series of 1,000 insanity, mental deficiency, and epilepsy were reported in the families of 86 cases and in another 26 there was a less precise history of familial neuropathic taint, which findings the committee believes are no greater than those to be found in the families of 1,000 non-criminal boys.

From Rüdin's institute comes a study by Stumpfl, who

[1] For an interesting but not very conclusive paper on the physical constitution of criminals, see Riedl, M.: "Ueber Beziehungen von geistigkörperlicher Konstitution zu Kriminalität und anderen Defekten"; Mnschr. Kriminalpsychologie, 23, 473-484, 1932. From Lombroso's time to ours efforts have been made to find a different sexual and obvious physical constitution for criminals. This effort has, in the main, entirely failed. See for a criticism of all this work the report of the Wickersham Committee, Ploscowe, Morris: "Some Causative Factors in Criminality" in the Report on the Causes of Crime, v. I, United States Government Printing Office, Washington, June 26, 1931.

concludes that more criminals are found among the relatives of habitual or recidivist criminals than among the relatives of those who commit but one crime. This is true not only of siblings brought up under the same or similar environment but also in the case of cousins reared apart. Thus, relatively more habitual criminals are found among the cousins of habitual criminals than among the cousins of such criminals who have broken the law but once.

Mayer stresses the importance of the affective factors in the attitudes of the individual to the outside world and especially in relationship to crime, but states that tests for detecting this affective disturbance are inadequate, which leaves the committee with this question, whence his ability to postulate that an affective disturbance exists?

Gillin is among those who agree that there is a much greater significance to be laid on social conditions and individual life experiences in the development of criminal careers than on hereditary factors and does not tend to believe that sterilization would be of importance.

Most writers agree that while there may be a constitution which in its reaction to the milieu appears as criminal conduct, the effort to breed it out by any eugenical measures is, in the present state of our knowledge not to be recommended, and that more fruitful approaches to crime are to be found in social measures of one type or another. Jennings quite eloquently states this to be the case and does not believe that the genetic approach to crime is at the present time of any practical importance and stresses this, that education, training, better health conditions, and better economic circumstances are the fruitful measures by which criminality is to be lessened.[1]

[1] Those who are interested in crime and its genesis are referred to the brilliant series of articles by Ploscowe in the Report of the Wickersham Crime Commission. The complexity of the problem and the flimsiness of most of the psychiatric, psychologic, and social explanations are delineated in a masterful and convincing way.

IX

TWINS

The characteristics of monozygotic and dizygotic twins have become critical in the discussion of the relative influence of heredity and environment in the creation and shaping of the physical and mental characteristics of man. We, therefore, make a special section of this important subject, including in our discussion, first, the nature and bearing of the general studies that have been done, and second, those which relate more especially to the question of the heredity of the mental diseases.

Since one of the most important compilations done in an objective way on the whole matter is that of Schwesinger, we abstract her presentation of the matter.[1]

Summary of Schwesinger's Critical Study

The results of the studies of twins . . . may be summarized as follows:

(1) There are clearly two types of twins, different in origin: "identical" and "fraternal."[2] Identical twins are of uniovular and monozygotic origin, and fraternal twins of binovular or dizygotic origin. The development of "identical" twins may be

[1] The most important workers appear to be Galton, Thorndike, Merriman, Lauterbach, Wingfield, Averill, Mueller, von Verschuer, Fortuyn, Bakwin, Lange, Rosanoff and his co-workers and Gesell.

[2] Since, as pointed out by Rosanoff, the term identical denotes something which is never present, complete identity, we agree that the term "monozygotic" is preferable, and as the opposite, the term "dizygotic" is substituted for fraternal.

influenced by the age when ovular or embryonic separation takes place, and by intra-uterine placement. About twenty-five per cent of all twins, and forty per cent or slightly more of all like-sexed twins are identical.

(2) Identical twins, selected on the basis of resemblance in physical traits, are found to be much more alike in test intelligence than fraternal twins, even than fraternal like-sexed twins. Correlation coefficients in the vicinity of .88 to .90 have been reliably established in the case of identical twins in contrast to the coefficients in the vicinity of .60 to .70 in the case of fraternal twins (Holzinger and Wingfield data). The average intra-pair difference in I.Q. as determined by the Chicago investigators is 5.3 in the case of identical twins, and 9.9 in the case of fraternal twins . . .

(3) In most studies no significant differences in intelligence are found between older and younger twins, especially between older and younger identical twins. The Chicago study shows more marked differences with age for fraternal than for identical twins. Apparently environment can be more effective in effecting differences where there is initial genetic variation than where there is none.

(4) The degree of resemblance in traits whose accomplishment depends on training is not noticeably higher than the accomplishment in traits not dependent on training.

(5) Gesell and his co-workers, by the use of co-twin control technique, have shown that training in the early years is highly dependent upon maturation of neural and muscular structure. This principle may be applicable to verbal as well as to motor training.

(6) Among the ten cases on record of identical twins reared apart since infancy, but coming together and objectively studied in maturity, there is, in six cases, no significant difference in tested intelligence: (a) "B" and "J" differ by three raw score points on Alpha; (b) "C" and "O" differ by two points on Stanford-Binet I.Q.; (c) "B" and "D" differ by four points on Stanford-Binet and almost none on other tests; (e) Richard and Raymond differ by one point I.Q.; and (f) Harold and Holden by six points. This agreement is the more striking because in one case ("B" and "J") there was much discrepancy in formal education, although possibly not in the cultural levels of the homes. This pair show superior intelligence. The pair ("C" and "O") had about equal schooling, and show ordinary intelligence. "B" and "D,"

Richard and Raymond, and Harold and Holden had almost equivalent schooling; while Ada and Ida, each having only a third grade education, both register normal intelligence. In two cases, twelve points difference in intelligence quotient is found between the twins, while the mates in the remaining cases differ by fifteen and seventeen points. A difference of this degree (12 points) or greater is found in ten per cent of the identical twins reared together in the Chicago sample and has been noted in other collections of identical twin data. In one case ("A" and "O") the twin making the lower score has a record of lower social status and malnutrition (in England, during the war), but schooling about equal in amount to that of the co-twin, although less academic in character. Her I.Q. is 84.9; her sister's is 96.9. In another case ("E" and "G") the twin making the lower score (I.Q. 66) had been kept home from school a good deal to help with housework. Her sister (I.Q. 76) had had an irregular, but apparently more favorable, nurture and education. In the case of "M" and "R" there were pronounced differences in cultural levels of the home; and in parent-child relationships which resulted in definitely different temperaments for the two girls. For Mabel and Mary the items of distinction were four years difference in schooling and rural versus urban residence. The lesser-schooled farm girl recorded 88.5, the urban and more educated twin 106.2 I.Q.

(7) To generalize on the basis of ten cases is not reliable, but a summary of these ten is permissible. The *average* of their intra-pair differences is 7.7 I.Q. points and the variability is from zero to seventeen points. These summaries can be compared with corresponding figures obtained on identical twins reared together, whose *average* intra-pair difference in I.Q. is 5.3, and whose *variability* is from 0 to twenty (or twenty-nine) points. These figures can also be compared with fraternal twins reared together, whose average intra-pair difference is 9.9 I.Q. points, and whose variability ranges from zero to forty-three points. They can also be compared with test-retest differences on the same individuals whose average inter-test difference is 6.8 points, and whose variability ranges from zero to fifty-three points.

Conclusions

By far the greatest interest attaches to a comparative study of identical twins reared together with identical twins reared apart; but until more data, accurate as to detail, are assembled on such twins separated in infancy, it is impossible to draw final conclusions on the effects of differences in environment on development of test intelligence. Workers must be cautioned against making deductions that, merely because the twins have been separated, their environments have been essentially "different." It is quite possible for two separate foster homes, having relatively similar standards and requirements, to be highly "similar" (e.g., as in the case of Ada and Ida). It is equally possible, on the other hand, for two different environments to obtain within the one physical home—as illustrated in the case of Esther and Naomi. To capture these subtle factors and operations of environment, rather careful measuring devices must be standardized and employed.

Such "measures of environment" are comparatively new, having only made their appearance within the last five years or so of socio-psychological research.

This introduces a second caution to the student of environment, namely, the need to guard against interpretations based on differences of group averages. Variability of test intelligence within groups is even more significant than their averages; a comparison of two sets of variation is as important as two sets of averages; and variability of one factor must always be studied with respect to variability of all possible influencing factors.

If the environments of separated pairs—individuals or groups—were rated quantitatively, new interpretations would be inevitable; and the *extent* to which *degrees of specific environment* corresponded with *intellectual variation* could be found. In the meantime, we have to depend, much less accurately, on social history reports based in large part on highly uncertain personal memory, opinion, and anecdotal account.

So much concerning the general subject of the characteristics of monozygotic and dizygotic twins.[1]

We turn now to the subject-matter of the psychoses, mental deficiency, epilepsy, and criminality in twins. The most important information is contained in the writings of Merriman and Rosanoff and his co-workers.

[1] O. von Verschuer, whose important studies merit especial attention, has gathered together important statistics on the high correlation existing in identical twins for physical characteristics. Especially interesting is the close correlation for the incidence and pathological character of tuberculosis in monozygotic twins.

We turn the attention of the reader to an important paper by Merriman on psychoses in identical twins, which we here abstract:

Sir Francis Galton in 1883 in his pioneer work stated "Twins have a special claim upon our attention; it is that their history affords us a means of distinguishing between the effects of tendencies received at birth and those that were imposed by the special circumstances of their after lives."

In this country, Benjamin Rush in 1812, in his book on mental diseases, cited a case of what was evidently manic-depressive insanity in two Revolutionary soldiers, identical twins, who were affected with "hereditary madness."

Since then, a number of instances of mental disease in twins have been reported, but usually the reports have failed either to state that the twins were identical or to offer proof that due observation had been made to establish their similarity. For example, the only report from the New York State hospitals was one by Smith, 1912, on several cases of concurrent insanity in twins, but there was no distinction made between fraternal and identical pairs. The psychoses appeared to be of the same type in what may have been two sets of identical twins and of the same type in a pair of unlike sex and therefore not identical. In his other cases there was available for study only one individual of each pair. A survey of the literature on psychoses in twins reveals a disappointing absence of a determination of identity or fraternity. It also fails to show, with four exceptions to be mentioned later, a report of a functional psychosis in only one in a pair of identical twins. More recently the literature shows a tendency to settle the question of identity, thus making the observations of value in this study.

It is estimated by Joseph B. DeLee in his "Principles and Practice of Obstetrics," that twins occur in 1 out of 87 births and that uniovular twins occur in 15.5 per cent of twin births. It is probable that the rates vary considerably among different races and at different times.

Data on organic nervous disease, not of exogenous character so far as known, were collected by Wilson and Wolfsohn, who claim that there have been few published cases. They mention epilepsy and Friedreich's ataxia and describe, as coming under their observation, cases of congenital nuclear ophthalmoplegia, cerebral diplegia and epilepsy. Regarding this last disorder, only one instance has occurred at Craig Colony for Epileptics in which any kind of twins were known each to be affected with the syndrome and in this case the twins were homologous, and an impression exists that no adequate study of data has been published. This disease may, so far as known, have more than one etiology, and freedom from symptoms in only one of an homologous pair would throw additional light on the problem, provided each of the two individuals was subjected to equal environmental influences, and the post-mortem brain findings did not show acquired pathology. Likewise, the problem of mental enfeeblement—many homologous pairs being known—is complicated by the fact that one member of the set may be impaired during birth delivery or afterward by injury or infection, both of which are recognized as factors in the production of mental defect, and yet are not always determined in the history of a case.

Mongolism has occurred in one of twins, which is consistent with its non-consecutive appearance, and this shows a probable absence of etiology in the uterine environment.

Resuming the consideration of psychoses in identical twins, Franz reported dementia praecox beginning in a pair at 20 years of age. Parker investigated this case further and satisfied himself that they were identical. He reported a second instance, the one developing insidiously from 16 to 19 years of age, the other apparently suddenly at 19, both receiving hospitalization at the same time but in different institutions. After 33 years they were both in the same hospital and it was noted that not only were their appearances sufficiently similar for them to be mistaken for each other, but their mannerisms were strikingly alike. Parker, director emeritus of Harvard University Zoological Laboratories, has recently written, in response to inquiry, that no further cases of the kind under attention have been learned of by him, nor has he been able to get evidence of a case in which only one of homologous twins had dementia praecox. He concludes that dementia praecox is germinal in origin.

Siemens, in his survey of the pathology of twins, collected seventeen cases of dementia praecox among them, six of which were undoubtedly in homologous pairs, five were doubtful and six were fraternal. He failed to find the disease confined to only one of an identical pair; and in three of the six identical pairs found the onset "simultaneous," in a fourth a year in separation, and in the remaining two doubtful as to the interval between onsets.

Newel reported a case of homologous twin sisters, one of which was partially paralyzed from infantile paralysis, and who, with the occurrence of the incapacity, developed a lack of self-confidence, seclusiveness, feelings of inferiority to and jealousy of her twin sister, particularly as the result of suffering comments of comparison unfavorable to herself. While she did not develop a psychosis, her temperament was modified to one of general suspiciousness and her intellect was inferior, perhaps due to the same unhappy comparisons, although the poliomyelitis, which occurred at the age of two, may have extended to the brain, as, in spite of the fact that she had walked a few months earlier than her sister, she fell behind her sister in learning to speak after the disease and while relearning to walk, and formulated sentences three years later than her twin. In this case there remains the doubtful element of brain damage at the time of paralytic infection.

Merriman himself adds a case of two female identical twins who became afflicted with schizophrenic disease at an interval of three years, one with catatonic dementia praecox, the other with paranoid schizophrenia. The author concludes from these cases and from the literature that dementia praecox or manic-depressive psychosis rarely occurs in only one of a pair of identical twins, this being a proof of their hereditary etiology.

We turn to the work of Rosanoff and his co-workers, whose studies deserve the widest dissemination not only because of the scope of the inquiry but because of the importance of the results. One objectionable feature which is usually found in the collection of cases has been eliminated in this study, that is, the material is unselected. The following is abstracted from his paper on the etiology of so-called schizophrenic psychoses, with special reference to their occurrence in twins:

The main object of the investigation in each case is two-fold: first, to determine the type of twins, that is, whether monozygotic or dizygotic, and secondly, whether the second twin, too, is affected by the condition in question, or by some allied condition or not at all.

A very interesting table is cited by the authors from Luxenburger in which this author "furnishes a number of tables in which he contrasts the results obtained by the above-mentioned three methods of collecting material: massing individual cases, reports of which are scattered in the medical literature, the questionnaire method, and the method of an uninterrupted series." For the reader's convenience we have reproduced his figures for schizophrenia in Table X. It will be seen that in the material collected by the first two methods 76.4 per cent of the ascertained cases were those of monozygotic twins, whereas in the uninterrupted series the proportion is but 36.2 per cent—a figure corresponding more closely to the proportion of monozygotic twins occurring among twins in general.

It will be seen, further, that among the cases collected by the first two methods both twins were reported as affected in 71.4 per cent of the cases, whereas in the uninterrupted series the corresponding figure is but 19.8 per cent.

TABLE X

Results Obtained by Three Methods of Collecting Cases of Schizophrenia in Twins (from Luxenburger, quoted from Rosanoff, Handy, Plesset, and Brush).

Method of collecting material	Monozygotic			Dizygotic			Type of Twins unascertained		
	Both affected	One affected	Totals	Both affected	One affected	Totals	Both affected	One affected	Totals
Cases from the literature.....	31	3	34	3	5	8	9	2	11
Questionnaire method.......	7	1	8	..	5	5	5	6	11
Uninterrupted series........	14	7	21	..	37	37	2	21	23
Totals................	52	11	63	3	47	50	16	29	45

The material of Rosanoff and his collaborators is contained in a table here adduced concerning which the authors state:

TABLE XI

New Cases of Schizophrenia in Twins (from Rosanoff, Handy, Plesset, and Brush).

	Same-sex twins				Opposite-sex twins (dizygotic)	Totals
	Probably monozygotic		Probably dizygotic			
	Males	Females	Males	Females		
Both affected.	10	18	3	7	5	43
One affected..	9	4	8	35	{21 (Males) 22 (Females)}	99
Totals...	19	22	11	42	48	142

It will be seen also that in 30.3 per cent of our cases both twins of the pair are affected. However, this figure includes dissimilar as well as similar affections. . . .

. . . The principal finding revealed by the table is a marked contrast between the monozygotic and dizygotic twins with respect to the proportions of cases of both twins of the pair affected. These proportions are, respectively, 68.3 per cent and 14.9 per cent.

The monozygotic twins tended to have similar affections. However, there are cases in which the monozygotic twins showed quantitative dissimilarity in five cases, and in one of them a qualitative dissimilarity in that epileptiform convulsions occurred, in only one of the pair.

The authors cite three cases as instances of qualitative dissimilarity. One patient had schizophrenic psychosis, the other epilepsy associated with mental deficiency. In the second case, one had a chronic schizophrenic psychosis, the other was an alcoholic. In the third, one had a schizophrenic psychosis, and the other simple mental deficiency. There are two cases submitted in which one twin has schizophrenic psychosis and the other is free from any neuropsychiatric condition.

Of the dizygotic twins, the authors cite cases in which they are similarly affected and others in which there is quantitative dissimilarity, both twins having the same psychosis. In a third case, one shows chronic schizophrenia and the other subnormal intelligence and a paranoid temperament. There are four cases in which of the dizygotic twins, one had schizophrenia and the other twin was normal.

The authors are developing a theory of the pathogenesis of dementia praecox in which environmental factors play a role and formulate the following general propositions in relationship to the heredity of dementia praecox:

1. In the etiology of so-called schizophrenic psychoses hereditary factors seem to play an important part.
2. The hereditary factors, in themselves, are often inadequate; that is to say, they do not suffice to produce a schizophrenic psychosis.
3. The pathogenic effect of the hereditary factors is not highly specific. Other factors often play a part with resulting dissimilarities of manifestation or total discordance of findings even in monozygotic twins.
4. Hereditary factors are not always present, therefore not essential, in the etiology of so-called schizophrenic psychoses.

These views coincide with those of the committee, and confirm the result of those researches which have been carried out on other than identical twin material.

We make a brief abstract of a paper by Rosanoff and his co-workers, entitled "The Etiology of Manic-Depressive Syndromes with Special Reference to Their Occurrence in Twins."

The authors studied 23 pairs of monozygotic twins, in which at least one of the pair had manic-depressive psychosis. In 16 cases both were affected, in 7 cases only 1 of the pair of the twins was affected. In definitely dizygotic twins of the opposite sex, in which at least 1 of the pair had manic-depressive psychosis and of which group 32 pairs were studied, it was found that 1 twin was affected in 29 cases, both twins in only 3 cases. This shows a definitely higher rate of affection of both twins in identical pairs. However, it is very striking to find that in more than one-third of the cases, manic-depressive psychosis did not occur in one of the monozygotic twins, the other being affected. That is to say, in less than two-thirds of the monozygotic twin pairs, manic-depressive psychosis occurred in both of the twin siblings.

The above findings are very striking, since they strongly indicate that while there is a constitutional factor operating, either an eliciting factor is necessary for the occurrence of manic-depressive psychosis, or monozygotic twins may be dissimilar in respect to the manic-depressive constitution. The latter interpretation seems unlikely; the former is, at the present stage of the problem, the preferable explanation.

Contrary to our expectation from eugenics but in line with clinical experience, the cases in which one monozygotic twin is free from manic-depressive psychosis outnumber the cases with corresponding results in dementia praecox. So far as twin studies are concerned, the result would indicate that dementia praecox is less related to environmental causation than is manic-depressive psychosis.

The bearing of the study of monozygotic twins on feeblemindedness is importantly exemplified by Rosanoff's paper on this subject. He finds a sex-linked factor in mental deficiency on the basis of an insufficient number of cases, there being 35 pairs of monozygotic twins and 60 pairs of dizygotic twins. There appears what was to be expected: in the case of the monozygotic twins, if one was mentally deficient, the other was in 33 out of 35 cases; whereas in 60 pairs of dizygotic twins, both twins were affected in 32 instances and only one of the twins was affected in 28 instances. When the dizygotic twins were divided up into sub-groups, same-sex and opposite-sex types, the following results were revealed: among the 33 pairs of the same-sex twins, both were affected in 21 instances and only 1 in 12 instances.

	Males	Females
mentally deficient	91	69
normal	10	20

However, it is quite evident that even 2 cases of monozygotic twins of dissimilar mental trends are of significance, either as indicating that monozygotic twins may have dissimilar constitutions or else that some environmental agent operated to produce feeblemindedness in the case of an individual by nature destined to be normal. Conversely, it appears that feeblemindedness is markedly linked up with constitution.

Rosanoff and Handy present further a complete series of all cases of Mongolism which occurred in at least one of a pair of twins, which were present in the literature and in addition 5 new cases. Altogether, they present the data on 27 pairs of twins, 5 of their own cases and 22 from the literature. Of these 27 pairs of twins, 6 were monozygotic and 21 dizygotic. In all of the 6 monozygotic twin pairs (1 their own case and 5 from the literature), always both twins were affected with Mongolism. In their 21 dizygotic pairs of twins, including some pairs of twins of unascertained type (4 of their own cases and 17 cases from the literature), only 1 twin was affected in 20 cases and only in one case both were affected. Rosanoff and Handy consider as an explanation for this very interesting fact that Mongolism may probably be a disease of the ovum itself, possibly due to abnormalities, such as scarification of the ovaries. They also find the incidence of Mongolism correlated to the age of the mother.

Although we adduce the above study, we believe that some explanations made are far-fetched. There is a considerable literature which shows that abortions, still-births, and general adverse development in utero is greater in the case of the male, just as the birth rate is definitely higher. It is not possible to link up this greater birth rate and greater lethality with any special factor nor with any special pathological condition. Moreover, while there may be a statistical preponderance of older mothers in the genesis of Mongolism, the cases of Broussard and those of Myerson show that young mothers, as a result of their first pregnancy, may produce Mongolian offspring.

Continuing their researches, Rosanoff and his co-workers considered the subject of epilepsy and its incidence in twins:

Summary: A general survey of 107 cases of epilepsy in twins is presented (in this paper). As regards the type of twins, these cases are classified as follows: monozygotic, 23; same-sex, dizygotic, 39; opposite-sex, dizygotic, 45.

The material was selected on the basis of at least one of the twins having epilepsy. The distribution of epilepsy and other neuropsychiatric conditions found among the other twins of the pairs is as follows: (1) in monozygotic twins, epilepsy, 12; deteriorating psychosis and tumor of the spinal cord, one each; normal, 9 (39.1%); (2) in dizygotic twins, epilepsy, 9; mental deficiency, 6; mental deficiency with psychosis, mental deficiency with behavior difficulty, deteriorating psychoses, behavior difficulty and dementia paralytica, one each; normal, 64 (76.2%).

Hereditary factors undoubtedly exist in the etiology of epilepsy as indicated by the comparison of monozygotic and dizygotic twins.[1]

The hereditary factors are often in themselves inadequate for the production of epilepsy, as is indicated by the large percentage of cases among monozygotic twins in which only one of the pair is affected.

The hereditary factors are not invariably present—therefore not essential—in the etiology of epilepsy, as is indicated by the high percentage of cases among dizygotic twins in which both of the pairs are affected. This point is revealed most clearly by a comparison of dizygotic twins, brothers and twin sisters with siblings of epileptic subjects; the percentage of those having epilepsy in the two groups, respectively, have been found to be 10.7 and from 1.1 to 4.1.

Identicalness of manifestations in both twins of a pair is the exception rather than the rule, even in cases of monozygotic

[1] The committee believes, in view of the writers' later remarks, that this statement should read: Hereditary factors undoubtedly exist *in some cases* of epilepsy.

twins as far as epilepsy is concerned. The dissimilarities in cases of both twins involved are quantitative (that is, as to the age of onset, frequency and severity of seizures, remissions, mental complications and outcome) and qualitative (that is, the other twin has no epilepsy but some other neuropsychiatric condition such as mental deficiency or psychiatric diseases). The dissimilarities are greater and more frequent in dizygotic than in monozygotic twins.

We do not follow the authors in their conclusion that hereditary factors are not essential because the incidence in twin dizygotic siblings is greater than in non-twin siblings. However, it is apparent that whatever constitutional factor is involved in epilepsy, it is less manifest and probably less important than in the case of the other disease conditions we have here considered, and that environmental factors, such as trauma, infection, and metabolic disturbance are to be sought for as eliciting and creating the epileptic manifestation.

A most important study on twins and delinquency is contributed by Rosanoff and his co-workers. They have collected 340 pairs of twins divided as follows:

Cases of adult criminality	97
Cases of juvenile delinquency	107
Cases of behavior difficulties in children	136

They then analyze this group of delinquents and criminals in Table XII.

There is a considerable point of difference between the results of the study of these authors and those of others (for example, Lange). They state:

We have in our adult criminality group 33 pairs of male twins which we have classified as probably monozygotic. In 22 of these cases both of the twins are criminal; and in 11 of these cases only one is criminal, the other not. This presents a contrast in comparison with the dizygotic male twins, of which there are 23 pairs in the adult criminality group. Here we find in only 3 cases both of the twins to be criminal; and in 20 cases only one is criminal, the other not. A similar showing is revealed by the female monozygotic and dizygotic twins, of which there are smaller numbers in our collection.

TABLE XII (from Rosanoff, Handy, and Rosanoff).

Type and Sex of Twins	Clinical Group		
	Adult Criminality	Juvenile Delinquency	Behavior Problems in Children
Same-sex twins, probably monozygotic:			
Males, both affected	22	25	21
Males, one affected	11	2	4
Females, both affected	3	14	20
Females, one affected	1	1	2
Same-sex twins, probably dizygotic:			
Males, both affected	3	11	13
Males, one affected	20	5	10
Females, both affected	2	9	13
Females, one affected	3	0	24
Opposite-sex twins, dizygotic:			
Both affected	1	8	8
Only male affected	21	28	18
Only female affected	10	4	3
Totals	97	107	136

The authors make a distinction between criminalism and criminality to the effect that criminalism is a strong and persistent constitutional tendency which manifests itself under various conditions of no special difficulty or strain, whereas criminality includes cases presenting an incidental maladjustment. (This differentiation seems to us to be a good one.) The authors go on to state that incidental criminality, as thus distinguished from criminalism, is more often found to affect only one of a pair of monozygotic twins.

They state that in the case of the juvenile delinquents, both of the monozygotic twins are more apt to be criminals than only one, but they make this pertinent remark: "This in itself is, of course, not conclusive of anything. It simply means that where we have similar heredity plus similar environment, then the behavior also may be expected to be similar."

They cite one instance of monozygotic twins reared apart who developed criminal tendencies at the same period of life, and despite the difference in environment. However, it is fair to say that they do not cite any great difference in environment. They merely state that one child lived with foster-parents who were very well-to-do and the other with a person who had fewer advantages to offer, which does not in itself indicate essential differences in environment.

What seems to appear from all this work on twins, so far as criminality is concerned is this—that under ordinary circumstances of life, monozygotic twins are near enough alike to respond in the same general way to the complex factors of the environment around them, and that some of them become criminals. However, even with nearly the same hereditary material, there is a very considerable proportion of different "fates" in this respect. One can speculate, as do the authors, in a complicated way, about hypothetical events which change the structure of the individual, either in the uterus or afterwards, and one may, properly enough, bring into the hypothesis such an unprovable conclusion as this one, that trauma may change the character of one twin and not the other. For the purposes of this report, however, all we can safely say is that there is, undoubtedly, an inborn constitution or temperament which, in certain instances, is definitely responsible for the criminal tendencies of the individual, given the kind of environment he lives in, but *that even in these cases there is nothing to show that this temperament would be handed down.* What needs to be studied in respect to criminals is (1) their marriage rate; (2) their prolificity; and (3) the fate of their children. None of the studies on crime and its relationship to heredity pays much attention to these important factors.

What has not been taken into account also in all the studies of monozygotic twins is this—that monozygotic twins come to constitute for each other a more intense social environment than the whole rest of the world put together, since they live in an intimacy with each other that is greater than even that of dizygotic twins and are linked together by a reciprocal attention of most potent quality. In other words, they tend to influence one another in a remarkable way; especially is this true of the earlier years of their life. Consequently, and independent of biology, they would tend to be alike in their attitudes toward life.

Summary of the Study of Psychoses in Monozygotic Twins

The literature bears out the conclusions reached by the committee in the previous pages. A very interesting fact is that the variability of the development of monozygotic twins is least with feeblemindedness, indicating that the hereditary or constitutional factor is by far the greatest in the condition or conditions of lowered intelligence. In criminality there is great variability, as is to be expected. What is rather surprising is that if one of identical twins has dementia praecox, the other is more liable to have a similar condition than is the case in manic-depressive psychosis. But while this difference is against the opinion expressed in the eugenic literature, it falls in line with the general clinical reaction to these two disease groups. The psychiatrist, as he deals with these conditions in his practice, *feels* that dementia praecox is, so to speak, deeply embedded in the nature of the individual, that there is a sort of fatalistic destiny operating. As he confronts the case of manic-depressive psychosis, he can feel a sympathy which arises from thc belief that here is a quasi-normal individual whose depression is in part a reaction to the melancholy phases of life and has some root in the harsh environmental realities.

X

GENIUS AND EUGENICS

The foregoing sections may be classified as the debit side of the inheritance of the psychoses, feeblemindedness, and epilepsy. Is there an asset side? Is there something to the aphorism of Dryden that great wit is to madness near allied? We need not subscribe to the extravagance of Lombroso and Nordau that genius is the far end of the polymorphic chain of degenerate characters which starts with idiocy. From Galton's work onwards there is accumulated evidence, the validity of which may be, to some extent, challenged, but which, in the main, is probably correct, that high ability has some familial relationship, that talent tends to appear in superior groups even though there are numerous exceptions where high ability springs up in the mass of the people in some measure, sufficient to reassure those who fear that talent and genius may die out because of the differential birth rate.

Terman's study of the gifted children of California throws some interesting, but not quite clear, light upon the situation. He states that gifted children are not only gifted in intelligence but also in character, especially in honesty and truthfulness. He believes that they show, on the whole, less psychopathic tendencies than the whole group, but this is based on the Woodworth test which has not yet been controlled by later following up the individuals tested. He shows, however, that there are numerous exceptions to the general rule with respect to character, personality, and emotional stability. He states further that the gifted are not free from faults and at least one out of five has at least more of them than the average children of the general population, and that one out of twenty presents a more serious problem in one or another respect. However, it may be stated that there is no evidence that these gifted children of Terman's really merit the term "genius." Certainly genius cannot be ascertained by the psychological tests of the present time, nor by progress in school, nor by any such criteria. A study of men of genius, in the real sense of the word, would probably show a few qualities that our present day psychological methods would not have discovered.

Turning to actual men of genius, that is, those whose careers entitle them to this appellation, is there anything to show that there is an unusual incidence of mental disease among their families and themselves? Lange-Eichbaum has done the most complete modern study on this subject, and while no conclusions can be drawn as to the general nature of genius, enough evidence is adduced in his work, which seems to us to be valid and reliable, to indicate that sterilization might readily cut off from the race some of its most valued and valuable members together with whatever effect it might have on the lessening of mental disease, feeblemindedness, and epilepsy.

Gaupp has dared to express this same belief in the New Germany, with special reference to the manic-depressive group.

While we may state categorically that feeblemindedness breeds no genius, and that we have nothing to fear on that score from the sterilization of the feebleminded, it does breed in very many instances, especially in the higher brackets, docile, servile, useful people who do the dirty work of the race, who are, so to speak, its servants, who might be unnecessary in an ideal system of society but who certainly fulfill a social function at the present time.

When it comes to the mental diseases, and especially manic-depressive psychosis, this may be stated—that in the clinical practice of everyday psychiatry, one runs into gifted individuals who are definitely hypomanic and for whom, in definite measure, the hypomania is part of the drive by which they succeed. Since no statistical evidence on this matter is obtainable at the present time, the statement is made only as an inference rather than a postulate. When one studies the histories of the men of genius as given by Lange-Eichbaum, one is impressed by the fact that many valuable members of society, worth more to it than the cost of maintenance of all state institutions put together, would have been lost if sterilization laws had been enacted on a compulsory basis a few centuries ago.

The following data are taken from Lange-Eichbaum's study.

Andersen, Hans C., (1805–1875): Grandfather and father psychotic, mother drunkard of masculine type, died from delirium tremens (Hansen and Moll).

Balzac, Honoré de: (1779–1850): Hypomanic psychopathic personality; his father had a depression for 20 years, did not leave his bed though not physically ill, then again took up his former life (Cabanes, Grasset).

Beethoven, Ludwig van (1770–1827): Paranoid psychopathic personality with tendency to abuse of alcohol. Father and grandmother drunkards.

Blücher, Gebhard L. (1742–1819): Prussian field marshal; hypomanic personality with deep depressions (1808, 1814, 1815–1816) in which also paranoid ideas occurred. In one depression he believed he was pregnant by an elephant. In his family many cases of manic-depressive insanity and suicide occurred. His great-great-grandfather in 1642 was decapitated for murder, another relative was decapitated for bigamy. One brother was a psychopathic querulent person. One son was insane. Blücher himself died in a depression with refusal of food (Haberkant).

Bonaparte, Napoleon (1769–1821): Father a neurotic hypomanic. Brother, Louis, definitely psychopathic. Sister, Pauline, hypomanic degenerative personality. Brother, Jerome, unstable. Napoleon himself neurotic, possibly suffering from rare attacks of affect-epilepsy and narcolepsy.

Byron, Lord George Gordon (1778–1824): Mother hysteric. Mother's father died by suicide.

Cardano, Geronimo (1501–1576): Physician and mathematician, psychopathic personality with hysteric, paranoic, and compulsive neurotic traits. His father was psychopathic, also his sons, one of them a criminal (murderer) (Rivari, Lombroso).

Diderot, Denis (1713–1784): One sister psychotic.

Dostoievski, Feodor Mikhailovich (1821–1881): Suffered from epilepsy. One son died in epileptic seizures.

Feuerbach, Anselm (1829–1880): Famous German painter. Hypersensitive psychopathic personality. His father (archaeologist) was autistic, depressive, mentally ill in his student years. Father's brother was schizophrenic. Another brother of his father (philosopher) was a schizoid personality.

Frederick the Great (1712–1786): King of Prussia. His grandfather, George I, and his ancestor, William the Younger, were schizophrenics.

von Goethe, Wolfgang (1749–1832): Sister a manic-depressive.

Gogol, Nicolai (1809–1852): Russian writer; father was a ne'er-do-well.

Grillparzer, Franz (1791–1872): Famous Austrian poet and dramatist. Depressive hypochondriac personality. Mother suffered from manic-depressive insanity (diagnosed as "mania menstrualis periodica"), died by suicide. One brother was suffering from a neurosis and from attacks of manic-depressive insanity. This brother's son committed suicide. Another brother died by suicide (Hinrichsen, Rank).

Hauff, Wilhelm: German poet and novelist. Mother suffered from "somnambulism." Mother's brother psychotic. Mother's mother melancholic. The sister of mother's mother had a psychosis. The son of another sister of mother's mother was the poet Justinus Kerner.

Hölderlin: German poet. Catatonic schizophrenia (developed after he had reached the height of his achievement). One great-nephew of his had an almost identical psychosis (Lange-Eichbaum).

von Kleist: German poet. Schizophrenic psychosis, committed suicide. One half sister, father's daughter, was restless, queer, masculine, finally developed psychosis. One cousin, melancholia, died by suicide.

Lenau, Nikolaus von: Austrian poet. Father psychopathic, mother hysteric, sister criminal (was in prison). Lenau himself developed dementia paralytica.

Mayer, Robert: Famous physicist, discoverer of the principle of conservation of energy, was suffering from manic-depressive insanity, usually hypomanic, with elations and depressions. He conceived his theory in a hypomanic state, while traveling in the South Seas. In 1850 attempt at suicide; 1852–1853 in insane asylum.

Michelangelo, Buonarroti (1475–1564): Father was suffering from periodic attacks of insanity with delusions of persecution.

Moerike: German poet. One brother querulent; another brother a ne'er-do-well.

Newton, Isaac (1642–1727): Psychotic from 50th year of life on. The psychosis was a late schizophrenia with incoherence, bizarre speech, depressive, persecutory and paranoid ideas.

Poe, Edgar Allan (1809–1849): Father a psychopathic personality. Mother a vagrant actress, died from phthisis of the lungs. One brother was a "half-crazy drunkard"; one sister an idiot. Poe himself was alcoholic, possibly on a depressive and epileptoid (dipsomanic) basis. He had attacks of delirium tremens. Since 1837 he was also taking opium and morphine.

Schumann, Robert (1810–1856): One son insane. Schumann himself was suffering from periodic attacks of an atypical psychosis with cycloid and schizoid elements. In between psychoneurotic personality. From 1850 on probably dementia paralytica. 1845–1850 increased production similar to Nietzsche. (Nietzsche is not incorporated in this group since he was suffering from dementia paralytica and there was no familial trait of endogenous insanity.)

Strindberg, August (1849–1912): Paraphrenia (paranoid schizophrenia) (Storch, Jaspers).

Swedenborg, Emanuel (1688–1772): Swedish philosopher, theologian and mystic. Late schizophrenia (paraphrenia) (Gruhle, Kleen, Jaspers).

Swift, Jonathan (1667–1745): Manic-depressive (Reid).

Tasso, Torquato (b. 1544): Famous Italian poet; schizophrenia with hallucinations and ideas of persecution.

Tolstoi, Lev Nikolaevich Count (1828–1910): Grandfather psychopathic (superstitious, gambler, borrowed money senselessly, undertook hundreds of things, ruined everything he had). Tolstoi himself was a depressive, schizoid psychopathic personality, with hysteric traits. He finally developed melancholia (Lourie, Freimark, Ossipoff).

Turgenev, Ivan Sergy (1818–1883): Psychopathic personality with pseudologia fantastica, finally psychotic (Radestock).

Verlaine, Paul (1844–1896): French poet. Vagrant, criminal, alcoholic, ethically defective; degenerative psychopathy with cycloid traits.

Wolf, Hugo (1860–1903): German composer. Manic-depressive psychosis; later developed dementia paralytica (Vorberg).

Bumke points out that the parents and siblings of manic-depressives, though having hereditary taint, which may express itself in their personality, are not sick people. On the contrary, they are frequently especially desirable members of human society, clever and efficient, active and full of drive, warm-hearted, and amiable, and sometimes geniuses. "If we would extinguish the manic-depressives from the world, we would deprive ourselves of an immeasurable amount of the beautiful and good, of color and warmth, of spirit and freshness in our lives. Finally only dried-up bureaucrats and schizophrenics would be left. Here I must say: I would rather accept in the bargain the diseased manic-depressives than to give up the healthy individuals of the same hereditary cycle."

XI

RECOMMENDATIONS OF THE COMMITTEE

THIS Committee has studied the principal literature of the world on the subject which was assigned to it by the Association. In many respects the survey has been disappointing in that it appears that not much scientifically valid work has been done on the subject of the inheritance of the diseases and conditions which have been considered. This might have been anticipated for neither psychiatry nor human genetics approach at present the status of exact sciences. It appears that most of the legislation which has been enacted so far is based more upon a desire to elevate the human race than upon proven facts.

We believe that certain definite, though in a sense negative, recommendations should first be made.

First. Our knowledge of human genetics has not the precision nor amplitude which would warrant the sterilization of people *who themselves are normal* in order to prevent the appearance, in their descendants, of manic-depressive psychosis, dementia praecox, feeblemindedness, epilepsy, criminal conduct or any of the conditions which we have had under consideration. An exception may exist in the case of normal parents of one or more children suffering from certain familial diseases, such as Tay-Sachs' amaurotic idiocy.

Second. Particularly do we wish to emphasize that there is at present no sound scientific basis for sterilization on account of immorality or character defect. Human conduct and character are matters of too complex a nature, too interwoven with social conditions, such as traditions, economics, education, training, opportunity and even prejudice, especially when these factors operate in the earlier years of life, to permit any definite conclusions to be drawn concerning the part which heredity plays in their genesis. Until and unless heredity can be shown to have an overwhelming importance in the causation of dangerous antisocial behavior, sterilization merely on the basis of conduct must continue to be regarded as a "cruel and unusual punishment."

Third. Nothing in the acceptance of heredity as a factor in the genesis of any condition considered by this report excludes the environmental agencies of life as equally potent and, in many instances, as even more effective. That scientific day is past when the germplasm and the environment are to be considered as separate agencies or as opposing forces. Both operate in the production of any character, though in different degrees, but the degree in which each operates is, at present, mostly in the field of the unknown. Neurology and psychiatry still have as their duty the laborious task of discovering pathology, pathogenesis and therapeutics even for those conditions in which heredity undoubtedly plays a role. Thus modern research has uncovered the fact that diabetes has a constitutional heredity basis. Yet the establishment of its relationship to the pancreas and the introduction of insulin are, none the less, triumphs of medicine.

We present the following recommendations concerning sterilization to the Association for its consideration:

1. Any law concerning sterilization passed in the United States under the present state of knowledge should be voluntary and regulatory rather than compulsory. The present survey clearly shows that the compulsory features of the laws which have been passed in this country have, with rare exceptions, remained unused. Either the custom of

obtaining the consent of the patient has become established, or the law has remained practically unenforced.

2. Any law concerning sterilization should be applicable not only to patients in State institutions but also to those in private institutions and those at large in the community. We see no reason for group or class discrimination.

3. The essential machinery for administering any law in regard to sterilization should be one or several boards composed chiefly of persons who have had especial training and experience in the problems involved, which should study each case on its individual merits, and should strongly urge, suggest, or recommend against, sterilization according to its findings. Cases could be brought before such a board by superintendents of institutions, private physicians, parents or guardians, or by the patients themselves. This arrangement would promote elasticity in the application of the law, and permit the utilization of future advances in knowledge.

4. Adequate legal protection for the members of such a board, and for the surgeons carrying out the recommendations, should be secured by statute.

Your Committee feels, in short, that it can only recommend sterilization in selected cases of certain diseases and with the consent of the patient or those responsible for him. We recommend that such selective sterilization be considered in cases of the following diseases (arranged roughly in the order in which sterilization would appear to be indicated):

(1) Huntington's chorea, hereditary optic atrophy, familial cases of Friedreich's ataxia, and certain other disabling degenerative diseases recognized to be hereditary.
(2) Feeblemindedness of familial type.
(3) Dementia praecox (schizophrenia).
(4) Manic-depressive psychosis.
(5) Epilepsy.

Each of these categories carries its own special implications:

1. Definitely hereditary and familial neurologic conditions are rare, but the indications for sterilization are usually obvious to the physician and should be so to the patient. The services of an expert board should be of value in doubtful cases.

2. There need be no hesitation in recommending sterilization in the case of feeblemindedness, though it need not, of course, be urged in the case of those conditions which are definitely of environmental origin. Though we hesitate to stress any purely social necessity for sterilization, it is obvious that in the case of the feebleminded there may be a social as well as a biological situation of importance. Certain of the feebleminded can only, under the most favorable circumstances, care for themselves, and a family of children may prove an overwhelming burden. However, in a world which has much low grade work to be done, there is still room for the people of low grade mentality of good character.

3. Dementia praecox will need, we believe, but little attention from the surgeon. Most cases which are recognized in time to prevent procreation spend their days in hospitals. Moreover, the sexual urge in dementia praecox is low and the marriage and birth rate correspondingly low. Those who come in contact with cases in the community or prior to their discharge from a hospital need not, however, in most cases hesitate to recommend sterilization since desirable qualities of other kinds are only incidental to dementia praecox and not part of its make-up. This does not, by any reasoning, apply to the so-called schizoid personality. There is no scientific proof to the effect that this personality type necessarily precedes the development of dementia praecox. Moreover those who are so labeled are often the bearers of qualities which make for great personal achievement and for the social welfare.

4. The problem of the manic-depressive psychoses presents complications which will tax the judgment of the

wisest board, and it must be met with conservatism and caution. The cyclothymic temperament is frequently the source of the highest achievement and ability of which mankind can boast. Decision in any case must take into account the total assets of the individual character as well as the liabilities incident to the psychosis.

5. The inclusion of epilepsy, in most instances, is mainly on the ground of the social situation rather than on its biology. If the epileptic attacks from which the individual suffers are infrequent and if the qualities of the personality are intact, we see no reason in our present knowledge for recommending sterilization. If the contrary holds true, then sterilization is desirable.

Further Research

The Committee believes that its most important recommendations are those looking toward a concerted, coordinated and planned long-time research. It is obvious to us that investigation of the problem of inheritance, especially of the psychiatric conditions, has been haphazard and often inexact. This is no criticism of the able men who have devotedly studied these most difficult problems and it well may be that no complete scientific approach is possible in the present state of our knowledge or rather of our ignorance, but it is time that a prolonged research be undertaken in which psychiatrists, statisticians, and geneticists will collaborate.

The obvious defects in the researches of the past may be summarized as follows:

(1) Control studies of the incidence of these diseases in the community are on the whole lacking. There is almost no knowledge of what may be called the psychiatric constitution of the community. Small samples have been studied here and there and mainly through the history and questionnaire method. Large samples of the population should be studied with personal contacts as the basis of the research. At least

ten years of organized effort would be necessary to obtain a background of facts essential for the proper evaluation of all work on the heredity of psychopathological conditions.

(2) The studies which have been conducted as to the incidence of disease in the families where ascendants, siblings or descendants of the patients in the hospitals have practically all depended upon the history method. Any experienced neurologist or psychiatrist knows how deplorably inadequate such a technique is, how replete with errors of omission and commission. It should be recognized that at least the immediate relatives of the patient admitted for the first time to any institution should be examined by an expert. This is especially urgent in the case of the feeble-minded, but the necessity for the collection of dependable data in other conditions is apparent. Any statistical analysis is not better than the data which it uses; one cannot make good sausage out of pork, old clothes and sawdust, no matter how good the mill.

(3) The coincidence of conditions, perhaps wholly unrelated, has too often been given significance in the studies which have directed the thinking in eugenics and psychiatry. To weigh the importance of the fact that a dementia praecox patient has an alcoholic ancestor, it is first of all necessary to know how the descendants of alcoholics, as a whole, compare with the descendants of non-alcoholics; and also whether the incidence of dementia praecox in these descendants is greater than that of the general population. So with other factors which prejudice or tradition may believe to be important as etiological either as a hereditary or blastophoric factor.

Your Committee, therefore, recommends that a permanent committee be appointed which shall take steps necessary for the organization of research in these directions. It may be necessary to interest a Foundation for the adequate financial support of a research lasting a decade at least. In the opinion of the present Committee, some State which is well organized psychiatrically and socially, and which has a stable population should be the scene of operations. A central group headed by a full-time director should determine, after due study, the techniques of research, this being the first and all-important step. Certain hospitals might be selected to study the mental diseases, feeblemindedness and epilepsy through the operations of a genetic group stationed therein. Arrangements could be made for the study of samples of the total population through schools, universities, factories, and such other institutions and social aggregations as may be decided upon.

With psychiatrists, psychologists, geneticists, and statisticians working together in a planned way, aided by the appropriate number of social workers and clerical assistants, the various problems relating to inheritance of neurological and psychiatric diseases might be clarified and the resultant knowledge become the basis of more appropriate action than is possible at the present time.

The Committee wishes to stress the fact which the diligent reader of the report will have noted; to wit, that in large measure marriage is a selective agency operating in a eugenic way. The barriers of marriage against unwise procreation might well be strengthened by appropriate and early legislation.

Furthermore, it is to be emphasized that no great or radical change in the complexion of society can be expected from any such sterilization program as we recommend, nor from any justifiable legislation. We do not believe that society needs to hurry into a program based on fear and propaganda. Although the problem of mental disease and defectiveness is enormous, there exists no new social or biological emergency.

REFERENCES

History of Sterilization and Laws

Gütt, A., Rüdin, E., Ruttke, F., Gesetz sur Verhütung erbkranken Nachwuchses. J. F. Lehmanns, Munich, 1934.

Holmes, S. J.: A Bibliography of Eugenics. University of California Publications in Zoology, 25, 1924.

Human Betterment Foundation, Collected papers on eugenic sterilization in California, Pasadena, California, 1930.

Landman, J. H.: Human Sterilization. The Macmillan Company, New York, 1932.

Laughlin, Harry H.: Eugenical Sterilization 1926. American Eugenics Society, New Haven, Conn.

Myerson, Abraham: A critique of proposed ideal sterilization legislation. Arch. Neur. and Psychiat., 33:453-463, 1935.

Peter, W. W.: Germany's sterilization program. Am. J. Public Health, 24, 3:187-191, 1934.

Popenoe, P. and Gosney, B. S.: Sterilization for Human Betterment. The Macmillan Company, New York, 1930.

Report of the Departmental Committee on Sterilization. His Majesty's Stationery Office, London, 1934.

Rossman, Mildred: Bibliography of legal articles on sterilization. J. of Hered., 26:88-90, 1935.

Siemens, Hermann W. and Barker, Lewellys F.: Race Hygiene and Heredity. D. Appleton and Company, New York and London, 1924.

Watkins, Harvey M.: Selective sterilization. Bull. Mass. Dept. Mental Disease, 16:3 and 4, 59-68, 1932.

Whitney, Leon F.: The Case for Sterilization. Frederick A. Stokes Company, New York, 1934.

We have personally examined the laws of the American states and of the foreign countries, and have communicated with the administrative authorities involved, whom we here take occasion to thank for their courtesy.

Main Arguments for Sterilization

Barr, Martin W.: Mental Defectives. P. Blakeston's Sons and Company, Philadelphia, 1904.

Bureau of Statistics, National Mental Hygiene Soc., State Hospital Press, 1922.

Dahlberg, G.: Die Fruchtbarkeit der Geisteskranken. Ztsch. Neur. 144, 427, 1933.

Dayton, Neil A.: Mortality in mental deficiency over a fourteen year period. Proc. 55th annual session of Am. Assoc. Study of Feebleminded, 204 ff. 1931. Size of family and birth order in mental disease. Publication of the Amer. Socio. Society, 24: 2, 1930.

Dept. of Commerce: Feebleminded and Epileptics in institutions. Bureau of Census, 65, 1932.

Dirksen, E.: Asoziale Familien. Deut. Ztsch. f. Ges. Pfl. I, 5 and 6, 7 and 8. 89, 129, 1924.

Elkind, Henry B.: The epidemiology of mental diseases, a preliminary discussion. Am. J. Psychiat. 6, 4, 1927.

Elkind, Henry B. and Taylor, Maurice: Unpublished paper.

Fernald, W. E.: After-care study of the patients discharged from Waverley for a period of twenty-five years. Ungraded, 5, 1919. Quoted by Myerson, A.: Inheritance of Mental Diseases. Williams and Wilkins, Baltimore, 1925, 81.

Human Betterment Foundation, pamphlet, Human sterilization. (This statement occurs in one form or another in the Collected Papers, Pasadena, California, 1930.)

Kende, Moritz: Die Entartung des Menschengeschlechts. Ihre Ursachen und die Mittel zu ihrer Bekämpfung. Halle, 1901.

Landman, J. H.: The human sterilization movement. J. Crim. Law and Criminol., 24, 3:400-408, 1933.

LaPage, C. P.: Feeblemindedness in children of school age. Manchester, 1911, 141.

Lenz, F.: Ueber die biologischen Grundlagen der Erziehung. Munich, 1925.

Mayer, Joseph: Gesetzliche Unfruchtbarmachung Geiteskranker. Studien zur Katholischen Sozial—und Wirtschaftsethik, 3, 1927, Freiburg.

Meyer, H.: Besteht bei vererbbaren Geisteskrankheiten, insbesondere bein Schizophrenie und manisch-depressivem Irresein ferner bei genuiner Epilepsie und Schwachsinn, eine erhöhte Sterblichkeit in dem Sinne, dass die Fortpflanzung der Kranken verringert wird? Allg. Ztsch. f. Psychiat., 100:48-61, 1933.

Myerson, Abraham: Inheritance of Mental Diseases. Williams and Wilkins, Baltimore, 1925, 109-113.

Myerson, Abraham: Researches in feeblemindedness. Bull. Mass. Dept. Mental Diseases, 14, 159, 1930.

Myerson, A. and Elkind, H. B.: Researches in feeblemindedness. Bull. Mass. Dept. Mental Disease, 14, 195-199, 1930.

O'Gorman, P. W.: Sterilization of the unfit. Med. Guard., 1, 96, 1923.

Pollock, H. and Furbush, Edith H.: Comparative statistics of state hospitals for mental diseases. State Hospital Press, Utica, 1922.

Pollock, Horatio M.: The depression and mental disease in New York State. Am. J. of Psychiat., 91, 4:763-771 (Jan.) 1935.

Popenoe, Paul: Fecundity of the insane. J. of Hered., 19, 2:80, 1928.

Popenoe, Paul: Social and economic status of the sterilized feebleminded. J. Applied Psych., 12:304-316, 1928. (See collected papers, no. xii.)

Popenoe, Paul: Eugenic sterilization etc. J. Social Hyg., 1, 27, 1928. (See also collected papers.)

Popenoe, Paul: Statistical studies of the patients of a psychiatrist in private practice. Am. J. Psychiat., 10, 125, 1930.

Report of the Departmental Committee on Sterilization. His Majesty's Stationery Office, London, 1934, p. 18.

Rüdin, E.: Studien ueber Vererbung und Entstehung geistiger Störungen. Monogr. aus dem Gesamtgebiete der Neurol. u. Psychiat. Julius Springer, Berlin, 1916, p. 45.

Statistical Bulletin: Mortality of patients in hospitals for mental diseases. Metropolitan Life Insurance Co., 19, 5: 2-3, 1928.

Statistical Bulletin, Metropolitan Life Insurance Co., 16, 2: 6-8, 1935.

Tredgold, A. F.: Mental Deficiency. William Wood and Co., New York, 1922, 169.

United States Government Printing Office: Mental patients in state hospitals, 1926 and 1927. Washington, 1930, p. 6.

United States Government Printing Office: Mental patients in state hospitals, 1928. Washington, 1931, p. 6.

Weinberg, W.: in Placzek's handbook: Künstliche Fehlgeburt und künstliche Unfruchtbarkeit; ihre Indikationen, Technik, und Rechtslage. Leipzig, 1918.

Winston, Ellen: The assumed increase of mental disease. Am. J. of Sociol. v. XL, no. 4, Jan. 1935.

Winston, Ellen: National Committee for Mental Hygiene: State hospitals in the depression—A survey of the effects of the economic crisis on the operation of institutions for the mentally ill, 1934.

Woodall, Charles S.: The children of mentally defective and mentally retarded mothers. Proc. of the 56th Annual Session of Am. Assoc. for the study of the feebleminded, held at Philadelphia, May 26, 1932.

Points of View Regarding Sterilization

Bruehl, Charles D. D.: The state and eugenical sterilization; Homiletic and Pastoral Review, 27, 1-6, Oct. 1926–Mar 1927; pp. 1-9.

Bruehl, Charles D. D.: The church and race improvement; Homiletic and Pastoral Review 26, 7, April–Sept. 1926, p. 903.

Davenport, Charles B.: Heredity in relation to eugenics; Homiletic and Pastoral Review, 27, 1-6, Oct. 1926–Mar. 1927; pp. 226-227.

Ellwood, Charles A.: The reconstruction of religion; Homiletic and Pastoral Review, 27, 1-6, Oct. 1926–Mar. 1927, pp. 571-572.

Gill, Frank A.: Sterilization of the unfit. The Lancet, 1:1380-1382, June 29, 1930.

Herd, Henry B.: Sterilization of the mentally defective. The Lancet, 2, 14:783-786, Sept. 1933.

Hill, Prof., A. V.: Sidgwick Lecture. Nature, Jan. 3, 1931.

Hobhouse, H. T.: Morals and Evolution. Henry Holt and Company, New York, 1906.

Lenz, Fritz: Menschliche Erblichkeitslehre und Rassenhygiene (Eugenik) v. 2, J. F. Lehmanns, Munich, 1932.

Mayer, Joseph, Gesetzliche Unfruchtbarmachung Geisteskranker. Studien zur Katholischen Sozial—und Wirtschaftsethik, 3, 1927, Freiburg.

Muckermann, H.: Kind und Volk. 6-105th ed. Freiburg, 1922.

Myerson, Abraham: A critique of proposed ideal sterilization legislation. Arch. Neur. and Psychiat., 33:453-463, 1935.

Pius XI: Reconstructing the social order. In Four Great Encyclicals, the Paulist Press, New York, p. 95-97.

Punnett, Prof.: quoted in article: Biology and eugenics; by Major Leonard Darwin, D.Sc., in Eugenics Rev. 13, 1:21-23, April 1931.

Report of the Departmental Committee on Sterilization. His Majesty's Stationery Office, London, 1934.

Whitney, L. F.: The Case for Sterilization. Frederick A. Stokes Co., New York, 1934.

Genetics and Its Relation to Eugenics

Adami, J. G. P.: Medical Contributions to the Study of Evolution. The Macmillan Co., New York, 1918, pp. 61, 151.

Harrison, J. W. H. and Garrett, F. C.: The induction of melanism in the lepidoptera and its subsequent inheritance. Proc. Roy. Soc. London, B. vol. 99, 241, 1926.

Hogben, Lancelot: The interaction of heredity and environment. J. Ment. Sci., 79, 590, 1933.

Holmes, Samuel J.: A Bibliography of Eugenics. Univ. of California Press, Berkeley, Cal., 1924.

Jennings, H. S.: The Biological Basis of Human Nature. W. W. Norton Co., New York, 1930.

Krout, M. H.: Heredity, environment, and developmental process. Psychol. Rev., 38, 187-211, 1931.

Morgan, Thomas H.: The Scientific Basis of Evolution. W. W. Norton Co., New York, 1932, p. 207-210.

Muller, H. J.: Artificial transmutation of the gene. Science, 66, 1927, p. 84.

Pearl, Raymond: Constitution and Health. Kegan Paul, Trench, Trubner & Co., Ltd., London, 1933.

Pearl, Raymond: Permanence and persistence of genes in the fruit-fly. Science, 81, 2100, Mar. 29, 1935, p. 8.

Plate, L.: Warum muss der Vererbungforscher an der Annahme einer Verebung erworbener Eigenschaften festhalten? Z. indukt. Abstammungslehre, 58, 266, 1931.

Riddle, Oscar: The control of heredity. Proc. of Third Race Betterment Conference, Jan. 2-6, 1928, p. 62-71.

Riddle, Oscar: Internal secretions in evolution and reproduction. Scient. Month., 26:202-216, Mar. 1928.

Riddle, Oscar: Some interrelations of sexuality, reproduction and internal secretion. J. A. M. A. 92, 12:943-950, Mar. 23, 1929.

Riddle, Oscar: The special contribution of developmental mechanics to the thought and purpose of the man of tomorrow. Proc. Am. Philosophical Society, 68, 2:107-117, 1929.

Riddle, Oscar and Bates, Robert W.: Concerning anterior pituitary hormones. Endocrinology, 17, 6:689-698, Nov.-Dec., 1933.

Rife, D. C.: Genetic studies of monozygotic twins. J. of Hered., 24:443-446, Nov., 1933.

Timoféeff-Ressovsky, H. A.: Induced gene-variations in Drosophila funebris. J. of Hered., 21, 167-171, 1930.

Verschuer, O. von: Neueste Ergebnisse der Erblehre und ihre Bedeutung für die Medizin. Z. orthop. Chir., 55, Beil. H., 9-26, 1932.

Vogt, O.: Neurology and eugenics. The role of experimental genetics in their development. Eug. Rev., 24, 15-18, 1934.

Watkins, Harvey M.: Selective sterilization. Bull. Mass. Dept. Mental Diseases, 16:3 and 4, 59-68, 1932.

Zeleny, C.: Genetics and embryology. Science 77:177-181, Feb. 17, 1933.

Studies on the Inheritance of Mental Diseases
Polymorphism

Beck, E.: Heredity factors in symptomatic psychoses. Mschr. f. Psychiat. u. Neurol. 77:38-70, 1930.

Brugger, C.: Zur Frage einer Belastungsstatistik der Durchschnittsbevölkerung. Ztsch. f.d.g. Neur. u. Psychiat. 118, 459-488, 1929.

Burr, C. W.: Heredity in epilepsy, a study of 1449 cases; Arch. of Neur. and Psychiat., 7:721-728, June, 1932.

Canavan, Myrtelle M.: The mental health of 581 offspring of nonpsychotic parents. Ment. Hyg. 7, 4:770-778, Oct., 1923.

Clouston, T. S.: Clinical Lectures on Mental Disease. 4th ed., Philadelphia and New York, 1897.

Déjèrine, A.: L'hérédité dans les maladies du système nerveux. Paris, 1896.

Diem, O.: Die psychoneurotische erbliche Belastung der Geistesgesunden und der Geisteskranken. Arch. f. Rass. u. Gesellsch. Biol., 2, 89, 1905.

Elderton, E. and Pearson, K.: A first study of the influence of parental alcoholism on the physique and ability of the offspring. Eugen. Lab. Mems., 10, 1910.

Féré, C.: La famille neuropathique. Paris, 1894.

Genil-Perrin, G. P. H.: Histoire des Origines et de l'Évolution de L'idée de dégénérescence en Médecine Mentale. Paris, 1913.

Jolly, P.: Die Heredität de Psychosen. Arch. f. Psych. u. Nervenkrankh., 52, 377, 1913.

Jolly, P.: Ueber Heredität bei Geistesgesunden und Geisteskranken. Med. Klin. 9, 364, 1913.

Koller, J.: Beitrag zur Erblichkeitsstatistik der Geisteskrankheiten im Kanton Zürich. Arch. f. Psych., 27, 268, 1895.

Krueger: Zur Frage nach einer vererbbaren Disposition zu Geisteskrankheiten und ihren Gesetzen. Ztsch. f.d.g. Neur. u. Psych., Orig. 24, 1914.

Lombroso, C.: Men of Genius. Walter Scott, London, 1891.

Luther, A.: Erblichkeitsbeziehungen der Psychosen. Ztsch. f.d.g. Neur. u. Psych., 25, 1914, p. 12.

Luxenburger, H.: Demographische und psychiatrische Untersuchungen in der engeren biologischen Familie von Paralytikerehegatten. Versuch einer Belastungsstatistik der Durchschnittsbevölkerung. Ztsch. Neur. u. Psychiat., 332-491, 1928.

McPherson, John: Identity of psychoses and neuroses. J. Ment. Sci. 66, 1920.

Morel: Traité des dégénérescences physiques, morales et intellectuelles de l'espèce humaine. Paris, 1860.

Myerson, Abraham: Inheritance of Mental Diseases. Williams and Wilkins, Baltimore, 1925.

Myerson, A. and Elkind H. B.: Researches in feeblemindedness. Bull. Mass. Dept. Mental Diseases, 14, 1-2; 108-229, April 1930.

Patrick, H. P. and Levy, E. M.: Early convulsions in epileptics and others. Arch. Neur. and Psychiat., v. 10, p. 715.

Pollock, Horatio M., Malzberg, Benjamin and Fuller, Raymond G.: Hereditary and Environmental factors in the causation of dementia praecox and manic-depressive psychoses. Psychiat. Quart., 7:450-479, 1933.

Riebeth, S.: Ueber das Vorkommen von Dementia Praecox und manisch—depressivem Irresein bei Geschwistern. Ztsch. f.d.g. Neur. u. Psych. Orig., 31, 1. 429, 1916.

Rüdin, E.: Studien ueber Vererbung und Entstehung geistiger Störungen. Monogr. aus dem Gesamtgebiete der Neurol. u. Psychiat., Julius Springer, Berlin, 1916.

Schulz: Zum Problem der Erbprognosebestimmung. Die Erkrankungsaussichten der Neffen und Nichten von Schizophrenen. Ztsch. Neur. u. Psych., 102, 137.

Stein, Calvert: Hereditary factors in epilepsy. Am. J. Psychiat. 12, 989, March 1933.

Wagner von Jauregg, Julius: Ueber erbliche Belastung. Wiener Klinische Wchenschr. Oct. 30, 1902.

Studies on Specific Mental Diseases

Davenport, C. B.: Heredity in Relation to Eugenics, Henry Holt and Co., New York, 1911.

Davenport and Muncey: Heredity factors in pellagra. Eugenics Record Office Bulletin, No. 44.

Schizophrenia

Alexander, Leo: Seven generations of a family with schizophrenic taint (in preparation).

Barrett, A. M.: Heredity relations in schizophrenia. Am. J. of Psychiat., 7:77-103, 1927–1928.

Bernstein, F.: Korrekturen bei erblichkeits-mathematischer Untersuchung von Krankheiten mit recessivem Erbgang. Arch. Rassenbiol. 27, 25, 1932.

Bleuler, E.: Dementia Praecox. Vienna, 1911.

Brugger, C.: Die erbbiologische Stellung der Pfropfschizophrenie. Ztsch. f.d.g. Neur. u. Psychiat., 113, 348-378.

Brugger, C.: Psychiatrisch-genealogische Untersuchungen an einer Allgäuer Landbevölkerung im Gebiet eines psychiatrischen Zensus. Ztsch. f.d.g. Neur. u. Psychiat., 145: 516-540, 1933.

Brugger, C.: Zur Frage einer Belastungsstatistik der Durchschnittsbevölkerung. Ztsch. f.d.g. Neur. u. Psychiat. 118, 459-488, 1929.

Diem, O.: Die psychoneurotische erbliche Belastung der Geistesgesunden und der Giesteskranken. Arch. f. Rass. u. Gesellsch. Biol., 2, 89, 1905.

Gengnagel, E.: Beitrag zum Problem der Erbprognosebestimmung, Ueber die Erkrankungsaussichten der Kinder von Schizophrenen. Ztsch. f.d.g. Neur. u. Psychiat., 145, 52-61, 1933.

Göppel: Untersuchungen der näheren Verwandeten von Allgäuer Reichsbahnangestellten auf Psychosenhäufigkeit und Kropbefallenheit. Gleichzeitig ein Beitrag zur Belastungsstatistik der Durchschnittsbevölkerung. Ztsch. f.d.g. Neur. u. Psychiat., 113, 455-478.

Hoffmann, H.: Die Nachkommenschaft bei endogenen. Psychosen. Julius Springer, Berlin, 1922.

Hoffmann, H.: Vererbung und Seelenleben. Julius Springer, Berlin, 1922.

Hogben, L.: The analysis of pedigrees. In: The Chances of Morbid Inheritance, C. P. Blacker, ed., William Wood and Co., Baltimore, 1934, p. 405.

Juda: Die Erkrankungsaussichten der Enkel von Schizophrenen. Ztsch. f.d.g. Neur. u. Psychiat., 113, 487.

Kalb, F. W.: Beitraege zur Belastungsfrage bei Paralyse. Ztsch. f.d.g. Neur. u. Psychiat. 70, 1921.

Kattentidt: Zur Frage einer Belastungsstatistik der Durchschnittsbevölkerung. (Die Erkrankungsverhältnisse in den Neffen—und Nichtenschaften von Paralytikerehegatten). Ztsch. f.d.g. Neur. u. Psychiat., 103, 288-306.

Koller, J.: Beitrag zur Erblichkeitsstatistik der Geisteskrankheiten im Kanton Zürich. Arch. f. Psych., 27, 268, 1895.

Kraepelin, E.: Psychiatrie, Leipzig, 1913.

Lundborg, H.: Medizinisch-biologische Familienforschungen innerhalb eines 2,232 koepfigen Bauerngeschlechts in Schweden, Prov. Blekinge, Gustav Fischer, Jena, 1913.

Luxenburger, H.: Demographische und psychiatrische Untersuchungen in der engeren biologischen Familie von Paralytikerehegatten. Versuch einer Belastungsstatistik der Durchschnittsbevölkerung. Ztsch. f.d.g. Neur. u. Psychiat., 332-491, 1928.

Luxenburger, H.: Erbbiologische Geschichtsbetrachtung, psychiatrische Eugenik und Kultur. Ztsch. f.d.g. Neur. u. Psychiat., 118:685-710, 1929.

Oberholzer; Erblichkeitsverhältnisse und Erbang bei Dementia Praecox, Zur 50. Jahres-versammlung des Vereins schweizerischer Irrenärzte, Genf, 1914. Albert Kündig.

Pollock, Horatio M., Malzberg, Benjamin and Fuller, Raymond G.: Hereditary and environmental factors in the causation of dementia praecox and manic-depressive psychoses. Chapt. III. Family stock of dementia praecox patients. Psychiat. Quart. 8, 3:553-599, July 1934.

Rosanoff, A. J.: Dissimilar heredity in mental disease. J. of Insanity, No. 1.1. Mendelism and neuropathic heredity. A reply to Dr. Heron's critique in Am. J. of Insanity, Jan. 1914.

Rüdin, E.: Zur Vererbung und Neuenstehung der Dementia Praecox. Monog. aus dem Gesamtgeb. de Neur. u. Psychiat., Julius Springer, Berlin, 1916, No. 12.

Schulz: Zum Problem der Erbprognosebestimmung. Die Erkrankungsaussichten der Neffen und Nichten von Schizophrenen. Ztsch. f.d.g. Neur. u. Psychiat., 102, 137.

Sünner, P.: Die psychoneurotische erbliche Belastung bei dem manisch-depressiven Irresein. Ztsch. f.d.g. Neur. u. Psychiat. Berlin, 1922, LXXVII, 453.

Weinberg, W.: Auslesewirkungen bei biologisch-statistischen Problemen. Arch. f. Rass. u. Ges.-Biol. 10. Jahrg. 417-451 u. 557-581, 1913.

Weinberg, W.: Die Kinder der Tuberkulösen. Leipzig, 1913, W. Hirzel.

Weinberg, W.: Ueber Methoden der Vererbungsforschung beim Menschen. Berlin., klin. Wchschr. 1912.

Weinberg, W.: Vererbung und Soziologie. Berlin, klin. Wchschr. 22, 14, 1912.

Weinberg, W.: Ueber neuere psychiatrische Vererbungsstatistik. Arch. f. Rass. u. Ges.-Biol. 303-312, 1913.

Wittermann, E.: Psychiatrische Familienforschung. Ztsch. f.d.g. Neur. u. Psychiat. 20:153-278, 1913. (See also twins.)

Manic-Depressive Psychosis

Banse, J.: Zum Problem der Erbprognosebestimmung (Vettern und Basen Manisch-Depressiver). Ztsch. f.d.g. Neur. u. Psychiat., 119, 576, 1929.

Blacker, C. P. (ed.): The Chances of Morbid Inheritance. William Wood and Co., Baltimore, 1934.

Brugger, C.: Zur Frage einer Belastungsstatistik der Durchschnittsbevölkerung. Ztsch. f.d.g. Neur. u. Psychiat. 118, 459-488, 1929.

Göppel: Untersuchungen der näheren Verwandten von Allgäuer Reichsbahnangestellten auf Psychosenhäufigkeit und Kropbefallenheit. Gleichzeitig ein Beitrag zur Belastungsstatistik der Durchschnittsbevölkerung. Ztsch. f.d.g. Neur. u. Psychiat., 113, 455-478.

Hoffmann, H.: Die Nachkommenschaft bei endogenen Psychosen. Julius Springer, Berlin, 1921.

Hoffmann, H.: Vererbung und Seelenleben. Julius Springer, Berlin, 1922.

Kattentidt: Zur Frage einer Belastungsstatistik der Durchschnittsbevölkerung. (Die Erkrankungsverhältnisse in den Neffen—und Nichtenschaften von Paralytikerehegatten). Ztsch. f.d.g. Neur. u. Psychiat., 103, 288-306.

Krueger: Zur Frage nach einer vererbbaren Disposition zu Geisteskrankheiten und ihren Gesetzen. Ztsch. f.d.g. Neur. u. Psych., Orig. 24, 1914.

Leonhard, K.: Atypische endogene Psychosen im Lichte der Familienforschung. Ztsch. f.d.g. Neur. u. Psychiat., 148, 52-562, 1934.

Luther, A.: Erblichkeitsbeziehungen der Psychosen. Ztsch. f.d.g. Neur. u. Psychiat., 25, 1914.

Luxenburger, H.: Erbprognose und praktische Eugenik im cyclothymen Kreise. Nervenarzt 5:505-518, 1932.

Luxenburger, H.: Demographische und psychiatrische Untersuchungen in der engeren biologischen Familie von Paralytikerehegatten. Versuch einer Belastungsstatistik der Durchschnittsbevölkerung. Ztsch. f.d.g. Neur. u. Psychiat., 332-491, 1928.

Myerson, Abraham: The Inheritance of Mental Diseases. Williams and Wilkins Co., Baltimore, 1925.

Paskind, H. A.: Hereditary factors in manic-depressive psychosis. Arch. Neur. and Psychiat., 24:747-752, Oct. 1930.

Pollock, Horatio M., Malzberg, Benjamin and Fuller, Raymond G.: Hereditary and environmental factors in the causation of dementia praecox and manic-depressive psychoses. Chapt. II. Do Mendelian laws apply to the inheritance of manic-depressive psychoses? Psychiat. Quart. 8, 2:337-371, Apr. 1934.

Rüdin, E.: Psychiatrische Indikation zur Sterilisierung. Das kommende Geschlecht, Bd. 5, 1930 (available in abridged translation as a pamphlet of the Eugenics Society).

Schulz: Zum Problem der Erbprognosebestimmung. Die Erkrankungsaussichten der Neffen und Nichten von Schizophrenen. Ztsch. f.d.g. Neur. u. Psychiat., 102, 137. (See also twins)

Feeblemindedness

Baker, G.: Mental and social status of 1500 patients in obstetrical clinic of Johns Hopkins Hospital; how this relates to problems of eugenics. Bull. Johns Hopkins Hospital, 52:275-314, April 1933.

Berry, R. J. A.: Mental deficiency. I. Some family histories of an unselected group. Eug. Rev. 24:285-288, 1933.

Berry, R. J. and Gordon, R. G.: Mental Defective. Kegan Paul, 1931.

Bielschowsky, M.: Amaurotische Idiotie und lipoidzellige Splenomegalie. J. f. Psychol. u. Neurol., 36, 103, 1928.

Brown, H. E.: The sterilization of the mentally defective. So. African M. J., 6:107-111; Feb. 27, 1932.

Brugger, C.: Zur Frage einer Belastungsstatistik der Durchschnittsbevölkerung. Ztsch. f.d.g. Neur. u. Psychiat. 118, 459-488, 1929.

Carter, A. D.: Case studies of mature identical twins. J. Genet. Psychol. 44: 154-174, 1934.

Clay, W. M. and Wilcox, E. M.: Five generations of an inferior family. J. of Hered., 18:121-123, March 1927.

Cordes, F. C. and Horner, W. D.: Infantile amaurotic family idiocy in two Japanese families. Am. J. Ophth. 12:5580561; July 1929.

Davenport, Charles B.: Heredity in Relation to Eugenics, Henry Holt and Co., New York, 1911.

Davies, S. P.: Social Control of the Feebleminded. The National Committee for Mental Hygiene, New York, 1923.

Dayton, Neil A: Influence of size of family upon the characteristics of the mentally deficient. Am. J. of Psychiat. v. 91, 4:799-832, Jan. 1935.

Dayton, Neil A.: Survey of retarded children in public schools of Massachusetts. Am. J. of Psychiat., 7:809-835, 1927–1928.

Dickey, L. B.: Mongolism in both of twins. Calif. and Western Medicine, 26, 346, March 1927.

Dietrich, H. and Berkley, H. K.: Mongolian idiocy; occurrence in twins; report of two cases. Calif. and Western Medicine, 24:498-499, April 1926.

Dunston, J. T.: The sterilization of the unfit. So. Afr. M. J., 6:112,117, Feb. 27, 1932.

English, W. M.: The feebleminded problem. Am. J. of Psychiat., 11: 1-8, July 1931.

Fisher, R. A.: Elimination of mental defects. J. of Hered., 18:529-531, 1927.

Freeman, F. N., Holzinger, J. J., and Mitchell, B. C.: The influence of environment on the intelligence, school achievement, and conduct of foster children. 27th Yearbook of Nat. Soc. for Study of Education, 1928, 103-218.

Goddard, H. H.: Feeblemindedness, its Cause and Consequences. The Macmillan Co., New York, 1923.

Gradle, H. S. and Folk, M. L.: Family idiocy. Am. J. Ophth. 10:6–602, Aug. 1927.

Herd, Henry: Inheritance of mental deficiency. Chapter 5 in the Chances of Morbid Inheritance, C. P. Blacker, ed., William Wood and Co., Baltimore, 1934.

Herrman, L. and Hogben, L.: The intellectual resemblance of twins. Proc. Roy. Soc. Edinburgh, 53:105-129, 1933.

Hill, H. G.: Heredity in cretinism. Simple and toxic goitre. Chapter 14 in The Chances of Morbid Inheritance, C. P. Blacker, ed., William Wood and Co., Baltimore, 1934.

Hirsch, N. D. M.: Twins: Heredity and Environment. Harvard Univ. Press, Cambridge, 1930.

Jacobi and Konstantinu: Quoted by Eyrich: Sterilisierung bei angeborenen Schwachsinn. Psychiat. Neur. Wchschr. 36, 373, 1934.

Jennings, H. F.: Biological Basis of Human Nature. W. W. Norton Co. New York, 1930.

Kufs, H.: Constitutional and hereditary pathologic basis for combination of infantile amaurotic idiocy with lipoid cell splenohepatomegaly. Ztsch. f.d.g. Neur. u. Psychiat., 117; 753: 765, 1928.

Kufs, H.: Identical pathogenesis of amaurotic familial idiocy and Niemann-Pick's splenohepatomegaly. Arch. f. Psychiat., 91:101-106, 1930.

Kühlmann, K.: Psychologisch-anthropologische Untersuchungen an Zwillingen. Jena Diss., 1932.

Lange, J.: Zwillingsbildung und Entwicklung der Persönlichkeit. Naturwiss. 1933, 94-100.

Lewis, E. O.: Quoted by L. S. Penrose in: Mental deficiency. II. The sub-cultural group. Eug. Rev. 24:289-291, 1933.

Lund, S. E. T.: A psychobiological study of a set of identical girl triplets. Human Biol. 5, 34, 1933.

MacGregor, R. R.: Case of amaurotic family idiocy. Canad. M. A. J. 16, 1362-1363, Nov. 1926.

Mohr, Otto: Heredity and Disease. W. W. Norton Co., New York, 1934.

Muller, H. J.: Mental traits and heredity. J. of Hered. 16; 12, 433-448, 1925.

Myerson, A. and Elkind H. B.: Researches in feeblemindedness. Bull. Mass. Dept. Mental Diseases, 16, 1-2:1080229, April 1930.

Newman, H. H.: Identical twins reared apart. J. of Hered., 20, 2:49-61, Feb. 1929.

Newman, H. H.: Mental and physical traits of twins reared apart. J. of Hered., 23:297-303, 1932.

Orgler, A.: Ueber Zwillingsbeobachtungen. Internat. Ztsch. Med. Psychol., 10:353, 1932.

Parker, P. A.: Variations in the mental development of twins. Proc. and Addr. Am. Assoc. Study of Feebleminded, 37, 213-221, 1932.

Pearson, Karl: On the Continuity of Mental Defect. Dulau and Co., London, 1914.

Penrose, L. S.: The complex determinants of amentia. Eug. Rev., 26: 121-126, 1934.

Reiter, H.: Effects of Anlage and environment in adopted illegitimate children. Klin. Wchschr. 9: 2358-2361, Dec. 13, 1930.

Report of the Departmental Committee on Sterilization. His Majesty's Stationery Office, London, 1934.

Rosanoff, A. J.: Sex-linked inheritance in mental deficiency. Am. J. of Psychiat., 11:289-297, Sept. 1931.

Rosanoff, A. J. and Inman-Kane, C. V.: Relation of premature birth and underweight condition at birth to mental deficiency. Am. J. of Psychiat., 13:829, January 1934.

Saleeby, C. W.: The Eugenic Prospect. Dodd, Mead and Co., New York, 1921.

Schwesinger, Gladys C.: Heredity and Environment. The Macmillan Co., New York, 1933.

Sontag, L. W. and Nelson, V. L.: A study of identical triplets. Part I. Comparison of the physical and mental traits of a set of monozygotic dichorionic triplets. J. of Hered., 24:473-480, 1933.

Stocks, P. and Karn, M. N.: A biometric investigation of twins and their brothers and sisters. Ann. of Eug., 5:1-55, 1933.

Tredgold, A. F.: Mental Deficiency. Balliere, Tyndal and Cox, 1929.

Usher, C. H.: A pedigree showing mental defects in four generations. Ann. of Eug., 5, 56-58, 1933.

Wildenskov, H. O.: Investigations into the Causes of Mental Deficiency. (Translation from Danish by Hans Andersen) Levin and Munksgaard, Copenhagen, and Humphrey Milford, Oxford University Press, London, 1934.

Wilson, P. T.: Study of sex-linked twins, twinning among relatives. J. of Hered., 21:371-374, Aug. 1930. (See also twins)

Epilepsy

Binswanger, Otto: Epilepsy. Nothnagel's System of Medicine, 12: 313, 1918.

Brain, W. R.: The inheritance of epilepsy. Quart. J. of Med., 29: 299-310, 1925–1926.

Burr, C. W.: Heredity in epilepsy. A study of 1449 cases. Arch. of Neur. and Psychiat., 7:721-728, June 1922.

Cobb, Stanley: Causes of epilepsy. Arch. of Neur. and Psychiat., 27, 5, May 1932.

Davenport, C. B.: Ecology of epilepsy. Racial and geographic distribution of epilepsy. Arch. of Neur. and Psychiat., 9:554-556, May 1923.

Davenport, C. B.: Heredity in Relation to Eugenics. Henry Holt and Co., New York, 1911.

Davenport and Weeks: Epilepsy. J. Nerv. and Ment. Dis., 28:64, 1911.

Davenport and Muncey: Hereditary factors in pellagra. Eug. Record Office Bull., No. 44.

Echeverria, G.: On Epilepsy. William Wood and Co., New York, 1870. (See also J. Ment. Sci. 1887, p. 620.)

Gaupp, R.: Die Unfruchtbarmachung geistig und sittlich Minderwertiger. Ztsch. f.d.g. Neur. u. Psychiat. 100:138-181, 1925–1926.

Gowers, W. R.: Epilepsy and other Chronic Convulsive Diseases. 1901.

Myerson, A.: Inheritance of Mental Diseases. Williams and Wilkins, Baltimore, 1925.

Oppenheim, H.: Textbook on Nervous Diseases. 6th Ed., Vol. 2. Epilepsy. Schulz and Co., Edinburgh.

Stein, Calvert: Hereditary factors in epilepsy. Am. J. of Psychiat., 12:989-1027, Mar. 1933.

Thom, D. A.: The frequency of epilepsy in the offspring of epileptics. Boston Med. and Surg. J., 175:573-575, Apr. 1916 and 175:599-600, Oct. 1916.

Chronic Progressive Neurological Diseases
Huntington's Chorea

Chapman, F. P.: Hereditary Huntington's chorea. J. Kansas M. Soc. 34:220-222, June 1933.

Popenoe, P. and Brousseau, K.: Hereditary Huntington's chorea. J. of Hered., 21:113-118, March 1930.

Riggenbach, M. and Werthemann, A.: Huntington's chorea in 48 members of one family. Schweiz. Arch. f. Neur. u. Psychiat. 31: 306-332, 1933.

Stone, C. S.: Huntington's chorea: sociological and genealogical study of new family. Ment. Hyg., 15:350-363, Apr. 1931.

Stone, S.: Chronic progressive chorea (Huntington's disease). New England J. Med., 207:974-983, Dec. 1, 1932.

Vessie, P. R.: Transmission of Huntington's chorea for 300 years, Bures family group. J. Nerv. and Ment. Dis., 76:553-573, Dec. 1932.

Worster-Drought, C. and Allen, I. M.: Hereditary Huntington's chorea, with report of 2 cases. Brit. M. J., 2:1149-1152, Dec. 21, 1929.

Acute Forms of Chorea

Cioffi, V.: Congenital chorea; case. Prat. pediat., 11:291-297, Sept. 1933.

Mikulowski, V.: Two cases of rheumatic chorea in one family and two cases of congenital syphilitis in another family. Rev. franc. de pediat., 9:386-396, 1933.

Schachter, M.: Acute familial chorea. Med. inf., 40:148-153, May 1933; also, J. de med. de Paris, 53:586-587, July 6, 1933; abstr., Hospital 21: 605-606, Oct. 1933.

Urechia, C. I. and Dragomir, L.: Congenital chorea; case. Bull. et mém. Soc. méd. d. hôp. de Paris, 49:1404-1406, Dec. 4, 1933.

Urechia, C. I. and Mihalesco, S.: Congenital chorea. Bull. et. mém. Soc. méd. d. hôp. de Paris, 50:1785, Dec. 30, 1926; also méd. inf., 33:34 Feb. 1927.

Athetosis

van Bogaert, L.: Hitherto undescribed type of familial diseases; myoclonus epilepsy with choreo-athetosis. Rev. neurol., 2:385-414, Oct. 1929.

Demerliac, M.: Case of double congenital athetosis. Rev. gen. de clin. et de thérap. 43:150-152, Mar. 9, 1929.

Oppenheim, H. and Vogt, C.: Wesen und Lokalisation der kongenitalen und infantilen Pseudobulbärparalyse. Journal f. Psychol. u. Neur. 18, s. 1, 293, 1911.

Friedreich's Ataxia

Baker, A. B.: Hereditary Friedreich's ataxia; clinical and pathological study. Am. J. Path., 10:113-124, Jan. 1934.

Giddings, G.: Friedreich's ataxia in 10 members of a family. J.A.M.A. 89: 1395-1397, Oct. 22, 1927.

Gordon, A.: Familial degenerative diseases. M. J. and Rec., 138:13-16, July 5, 1933.

Jones, A. B.: Hereditary ataxia: M. Clin. North America, 11:343-344, Sept. 1927.

Naffziger, H. C. and Shephardson, H. C.: New family group of hereditary and spastic ataxia; its distribution in California; preliminary report. Calif. and West. Med., 26:207-208, Feb. 1927.

Spastic Spinal Paralysis

Curtius, F.: Familial diffuse sclerosis and familial spastic paralysis in tribe; significance with regard to genealogy of heredodegenerations. Ztsch. f.d.g. Neur. u. Psychiat., 126:209-227, 1930.

Klein, R.: Heredity in familial spastic paralysis. Mnschr. f. Psychiat. u. Neur., 72:24-36, April 1929.

Schaffer, K.: Zur Pathologie und pathologischen Histologie der spastischen Heredo-degeneration (hereditäre spastische Spinal-paralyse). Deut. Ztsch. f. Nervenh. 73:101; 1922.

Worster-Drought, C., Hill, T. R. and McMenemey, W. H.: Spastic spinal paralysis with familial presenile dementia. J. Neur. and Psychopath., 14:27-34, July 1933.

Progressive Muscular Atrophy

Cavanaugh, W. J. and Tucker, H.: Progressive neural muscular atrophy; clinical report of 2 cases in brothers associated with mental symptoms. New Orleans M. and S. J., 81:290-293, Oct. 1928.

Gordon, I.: Muscular atrophy in 5 generations. Lancet, 2:1026-1029, Nov. 4, 1933.

Worster-Drought, C.: Unusual form of familial myopathy in a mother and two children. Proc. Roy. Soc. Med. 25:1540-1542, Aug. 1932.

Muscular Dystrophy

Kostakow, S.: Hereditary transmission and therapy with glycine. Klin. Wchnschr., 13:219-221, Feb. 10, 1934.

Minkowski, M. and Sidler, A.: Clinical and heredobiologic study of heredity in progressive muscular dystrophy Schweizer medizinische. Wchnschr., 58; 1005-1009, Oct. 13, 1928.

Monrad-Krohn, G. H.: Dystrophy in two brothers, whose father presented rudimentary myopathic affection of one limb only. Acta Psychiat. et. Neurol. 5:127, 1930.

Weitz, W.: Heredity of progressive muscular dystrophy. Deut. Ztsch. f. Nervenh. 102:209-220, 1928. (Comment on Diehl, Hansen and Ubisch's article.)

Myotonia (Thomsen's Disease)

Barker, L. F.: A case of congenital myotonia. M. Clin. North America 14:127-130, July 1930.

Böe, Gunnar: Myotonia congenita und Myotonia atrophica bei zwei Brüdern. Acta Med. scand. suppl. 50:128-139, 1932.

Burke, M. R.: Myotonia atrophica; case. J. Roy. Army M. Corps; 61:222-223, Sept. 1933.

Dias, Valdes R.: Ueber Thomsen'sche Krankheit. Arch. med. inf. hosp. Garia, 1, 15-33, 1932.

Elkington, J. H. C.: Two brothers affected with dystrophia myotonica. Proc. roy. soc. Med. 24, 315, 1931.

Ruhemann, K.: Myotonia congenita (Thomsen'sche Krankheit) und Betriebsunfall. Mnschr. f. Unfallheilkunde, 39: 445-456, 1932.

Urechia, O. T. Retezeanu, and Dragomir, L.: Paramyotonie congenitale. Troubles dans les échanges du calcium sanguin. Traitment par la parathyroide Richter. Bull. Soc. méd. hôp. Paris, III, 3. 48: 1430-1433, 1932.

Syringomyelia

Kino, F.: Hereditary familial syringomyelia; topical segmentation in cross-section of anterior horn. Ztsch. f.d.g. Neur. u. Psychiat., 107: 1-15, 1927.

Ostertag, B.: Syringomyelia, heredity. Verhandl. d. deutsch. path. Gesellsch., 25:166-174, 1930.

Ostertag, B.: Hereditary syringomyelia in rabbits. Deut. Ztsch. f. Nervenh. 117-119: 371-408, 1931.

Tenner, J.: Syringomyelia in father and daughter. Deut. Ztschr. f. Nervenh., 106: 13-25, 1928.

Wagner, I.: Familial lumbo-sacral syringomyelia. Mnschr. f. Kinderh. 53: 137-152, 1932.

Infantile Diplegia and Monoplegia

Baumann, C.: Eine besondere Form halbseitiger zentraler Kinderlaehmung. Psychiat. Bl., 36: 419-432, 1932.

Denzer, B. S.: Familial cerebral diplegia; heredodegenerative disease of the nervous system. Arch. of Pediat., 49, 693-697, 1932.

Paroxysmal Paralysis

Safran, M.: Ein Fall von familiärer paroxysmaler Paralyse. Sovrem. Psychoneur., 9:810-811, 1929.

Strauss, Hans: Zur Kasuistik der paroxysmalen Lähmung. Deutsche med. Wchnsch., 58, 1408, 1932.

Hereditary Optic Atrophy (Leber's Disease)

Ferguson, F. R. and Critchley, M.: Leber's optic atrophy and its relationship with heredo-familial ataxias. J. Neur. and Psychopath. 9:120-132, Oct. 1928.

Kuhn, H. C.: Hereditary optic atrophy (Leber's disease). A clinico-surgical study of a case. Arch. Ophthalm., 5, 408-417, 1931.

Merritt, H. Houston: Hereditary optic atrophy (Leber's disease). Arch. of Neur. and Psychiat., 24:775-781, 1930.

Diseases of the Peripheral Nerves

Castellino, P. G.: Familial neurofibromatosis; clinical and pathogenetic contribution Urol. and Cutan. Rev., 34, 384-390, June, 1930.

Frets, G. P.: Neurofibromatosis; hereditary aspect of 5 cases. Genetica, 11:347-366, 1928–1929.

Gerli, P.: Familial Neurofibromatosis; Clin. med. ital., 62:67-92, Jan., 1931.

Heine, L.: Zwei Doppelfaelle von Tumor des Kleinhirn-Brueckenwinkels mit und ohne Neurofibromatose. Ztsch. f.d.g. Neur. u. Psych. 100, 481, 1926.

Lazarescu, D. and E.: Recklinghausen's disease in mother and plexiform, palpebro-orbital neuroma in offspring. Ann. d'ocul. 168:166-186, Mar. 1931.

Struwe, F. and Steuer, E. J.: Neurofibromatosis; familial occurrence; clinical and anatomic study. Ztsch. f. d. g. Neur. u. Psychiat. 125: 748-790, 1930.

Zurid, I.: Ein Fall erblicher Vulnerabilität des peripherischen Nervensystems. Soviet. Nevropat., 1,219, 1932.

Crime

Creutz, W.: Der Einfluss der erblichen Belastung und der Umwelt bei Criminellen. Allg. Z. Psychiat., 95:73-106, 1931.

East, W. N.: Heredity and crime. Eug. Rev., 20:169-172, Oct. 1928.

Gillin, J. L.: Die Unfruchtbarmachung von Verbrechern. Mnschr. f. Krimpsychol. u. Strafrechtsref., 24:9-15, 1932.

Gruhle, E. W.: Vererbungsgesetze und Verbrechensbekämpfung. Mnschr. f. Krimpsychol. u. Strafrechtsref. 23:559-568, 1932.

Heimberger, Joseph: Strafkolonien. Neue Zeit u. Streitfragen; 3:67-95, 1906.

Jennings, H. S.: The Biological Basis of Human Nature. W. W. Norton Co., New York, 1930.

Lange, J.: Verbrechen und Vererbung. Eug. I., 165, 1931.

Lange, J.: Verbrechen als Schicksal. Leipzig, 1929. (English translation: Crime and Destiny. Boni, New York, 1930.)

Leavitt, F. H.: Psychiatry and the Criminal. Am. J. of Psychiat., 12: 541-554, 1932.

Legras, A. M.: Psychose und Kriminalität bei Zwillingen. Utrecht Diss. 1932.

Maier, B.: Ueber das Gemüt. Zentbl. f. Psychotherap., 5:333-343, 1932.

Mayer, Joseph: Gesetzliche Unfruchtbarmachung Geisteskranker. Herder and Co., Freiburg, 1927.

Ploscowe, Morris: Causes of Crime, in: Wickersham Committee Report, 1930.

Rüdin, E.: Ztsch. f. d. g. Neur. und Psychiat. vol. 514, 1924.

Sticker, G.: Geschlechtsleben und Fortpflanzung vom Standpunkt des Arztes. M. Gladbach, 1916.

Stumpfl, F.: Erbanlage und Verbrechen. I. Teil, Die Kriminalität bei den Geschwistern und bei den Vettern und Basen der Ausgangsfälle. Ztsch. f. d. g. Neur. u. Psychiat., 145:283-326, 1933.

Twins

Fortuyn, A. B. Droogleever: Modern research on human twins. Quart. Rev. of Biol., 7, 3:298-306 (Sept.), 1932.

Merriman, W. E.: Psychoses in identical twins. Psychiat. Quart., 7, 37-49, 1933.

Newell, H. W.: Differences in personalities in the surviving pair of identical triplets. Am. J. of Orthopsychiat., I, 61-80, 1930.

Rosanoff, A. J.: Sex-linked inheritance in mental deficiency. Am. J. of Psychiat., 11:289 (Sept.), 1931.

Rosanoff, A. J., and Handy, L. M.: The etiology of Mongolism with special reference to its occurrence in twins. Am. J. Dis. of Children, 48:764-779 (Oct.), 1934.

Rosanoff, A. J., Handy, L. M., and Plesset, I. R.: The etiology of manic-depressive syndromes with special reference to their occurrence in twins. Am. J. of Psychiat., 91, 4:725-761 (Jan.), 1935.

Rosanoff, A. J., Handy, L. M., Plesset, I. R., and Brush, S.: The etiology of so-called schizophrenic psychoses with special reference to their occurrence in twins. Am. J. of Psychiat. (Sept.), 1934.

Rosanoff, A. J., Handy, L. M., and Rosanoff, I. A.: Etiology of epilepsy with special reference to its occurrence in twins. Arch. of Neurol. and Psychiat., 31:1165 (June), 1934.

Rosanoff, A. J., Handy, L. M., and Rosanoff, I. A.: Criminality and delinquency in twins. J. Crimin. Law and Criminol., 24:923 (Jan.–Feb.) 1934.

Schwesinger, Gladys C.: Heredity and Environment. The Macmillan Co., New York, 1933.

Verschuer, O. von: Die Aehnlichkeitsdiagnose der Eineiigkeit von Zwillingen. Anthropologischer Anzeiger, 5, 244-248, 1928.

Verschuer, O. von: Die Variabilität des menschlichen Körpers an Hand von Wachstumsstudien an ein-und zweieiigen Zwillingen. Ztschr. für indukt. Abstammungs-und Vererbungslehre, Suppl. II, 1508-1516, 1928.

Verschuer, O. von: Erbbiolologische Untersuchungen an Zwillingen. Ztschr. f. indukt. Abstammungs und Vererbungslehre, 54:280-285, 1930.

Verschuer, O. von: Demonstrationen zur Zwillingsanthropologie. Verhandlungen der Gesellschaft für physische Anthropologie, 67-74, 1930.

Verschuer, O. von: Ergebnisse der Zwillingsforschung. Verhandlungen der Gesellschaft für physische Anthropologie, 6:1-65, 1931.

Genius and Eugenics

Becker: Denkwuerdigkeiten aus der Erbgeschichte. Psychiat. Neur. Wchschr. 36, 390, 1934.

Bumke, O.: Discussion to the paper of Faltlhauser: "Zur Frage der Sterilisierung geistig Abnormer," 25. Jahresversammlung des Vereins Bayerischer Psychiater, in Munich, July 18th and 19th, 1931; Allg. Ztsch. f. Psychiat. 96:372, 1932.

Gaupp, R.: Das Gesetz zur Verhütung erbkranken Nachwuchses und die Psychiatrie. Klim. Wchschr. I, 1, Jan. 1934.

Lange-Eichbaum, W.: Genie, Irsinn und Ruhm. Munich, 1928.

Lombroso, C.: Men of Genius. Walter Scott, London, 1891.

Popenoe, P.: Wird dein Sohn ein Genie sein? Eugenik I: 106-113, 1931.

Roesle, E.: Die Messung der Häufigkeit der Intelligenz bei den Ahnen von Hermann Grimm und Wolfgang Goethe als Beispiel für die praktische Auswertung von Ahnentafeln. Arch. soz. Hyg. 7:283, 1932.

Rossman, J.: Heredity and invention. J. of Hered. 21:507-512, Dec. 1930.

Terman, L. M.: Genetic Studies of Genius. Vol. I. Mental and Physical Traits of a Thousand Gifted Children. Stanford University Press, Stanford Univ., California, 1926.

AUTHOR INDEX

A

Adami, 75, 187
Alexander, 106, 190
Allen, 145, 198

B

Banse, 192
Baker, 193, 198
Barker, 184, 199
Barr, 55, 185
Barrett, 82, 99, 100, 190
Bates, 188
Baumann, 148, 200
Baur, 25
Beck, 88, 188
Becker, 203
Berkley, 113, 194
Bernstein, 190
Berry, 193
Bielschowsky, 114, 194
Binswanger, 137, 196
Blacker, 192
Bleuler, 99, 190
Böe, 148, 199
van Bogaert, 146, 148, 198
Brain, 139, 196
Brousseau, 197
Brown, 194
Bruehl, 187
Brugger, 46, 84, 101, 106, 107, 117, 189, 190, 192, 194
Brush, 160, 161, 202
Bumke, 175, 203
Burke, 148, 200
Burr, 86, 189, 196

C

Calverton, 2
Canavan, 87, 88, 189
Carter, 194
Castellino, 201
Castle, 71
Cavanaugh, 147
Chapman, 145, 197
Cioffi, 198
Clay, 194
Clouston, 82, 189
Cobb, 86, 141, 197
Cordes, 114, 194
Creutz, 201
Critchley, 149, 200
Curtius, 199

D

Dahlberg, 43, 185
Darwin, 2
Davenport, 83, 88, 90, 92, 118, 137, 141, 145, 187, 190, 194, 197
Davies, 194
Dayton, 48, 49, 50, 54, 122, 127, 142, 185, 194
Déjérine, 82, 189
Demerliac, 198
Denzer, 148, 200
Dias, 148, 200
Dickey, 194
Diem, 84, 118, 189, 191
Dietrich, 113, 194
Dirkson, 40, 185
Dragomir, 200
Dunston, 194

E

East, 151, 201
Echeverria, 197
Elderton, 87, 118, 142, 189
Elkind, 28, 30, 31, 32, 33, 47, 125, 185, 186, 189
Elkington, 148, 200
Ellwood, 64, 187
English, 194
Esquirol, 88

F

Féré, 82, 83, 189
Ferguson, 149, 200

Fernald, 44, 185
Fischer, 25
Fisher, 194
Folk, 114, 194
Forel, 3, 75
Fortuyn, 202
Freeman, 116, 133, 194
Frets, 201
Fuller, 101, 104, 111, 190, 192, 193
Furbush, 27, 142, 186

G

Galton, 2, 64, 170
Garrett, 187
Gaupp, 171, 197, 203
Gengnagel, 191
Genil-Perrin, 88, 189
Gerli, 201
Giddings, 146, 198
Gill, 187
Gillin, 152, 201
Goddard, 194
Goeppel, 101, 107, 191, 192
Gordon, 146, 147, 193, 198
Gosney, 5, 10, 184
Gowers, 137, 197
Gradle, 114, 194
Gruhle, 201
Guett, 184

H

Haldane, 71
Handy, 160, 161, 164, 167, 202
Harrison, 78, 187
Heimberger, 151, 201
Heine, 201
Herd, 65, 187, 195
Herrman, 195
Hill, 64, 113, 187, 195
Hirsch, 195
Hobhouse, 64, 187
Hoffmann, 75, 76, 92, 96, 108, 109, 110, 191, 192, 193
Hogben, 76, 187, 191
Holmes, O. W., 5
Holmes, S. J., 184, 187
Holzinger, 116, 133, 194
Horner, 114, 194

I

Inman-Kane, 131, 196

J

Jacobi, 113, 195
Jennings, 71, 152, 188, 195, 201
Jolly, 85, 189
Jones, 198
Juda, 106, 191

K

Kalb, 191
Karn, 196
Kattentidt, 101, 107, 191, 193
Kende, 25, 185
Klein, 199
Kino, 200
Koller, 84, 189, 191
Konstantinu, 113, 195
Kostakow, 199
Kraepelin, 99, 191
Kretschmer, 78, 107
Krout, 188
Krueger, 88, 189, 193
Kuehlmann, 195
Kufs, 114, 195
Kuhn, 149, 201

L

Landman, 24, 184, 185
Lange, 150, 166, 195, 201
Lange-Eichbaum, 172, 203
LaPage, 55, 185
Laughlin, 25, 184
Lazarescu, 201
Leavitt, 201
Legras, 201
Lenz, 25, 40, 60, 185, 187
Leonhard, 193
Levy, 86, 91, 190
Lewis, 114, 195
Lombroso, 82, 88, 170, 189, 203
Lund, 195
Lundborg, 90, 91, 92, 191
Luther, 88, 189, 193
Luxenburger, 84, 92, 101, 106, 107, 108, 110, 160, 189, 191, 193

M

MacGregor, 195
MacPherson, 82, 189
Maier, 202
Malzberg, 101, 104, 111, 190, 192, 193
Mayer, 25, 61, 62, 63, 151, 152, 185, 187, 202
Merriman, 157, 202
Merritt, 149, 201
Meyer, 53, 79, 185
Mikulowski, 198
Minkowski, 199

Mitchell, 116, 133, 194
Mjoen, 25
Mohr, 195
Monrad-Krohn, 147, 199
Morel, 82, 88, 189
Morgan, 70, 71, 188
Muckermann, 187
Muller, 78, 188, 195
Muncey, 190, 197
Myerson, 41, 47, 56, 59, 80, 81, 86, 88, 113, 117, 124, 125, 142, 184, 185, 186, 187, 189, 193, 195, 197

N

Naffziger, 146, 198
Nelson, 196
Newell, 202
Newman, 195
Nordau, 82, 170

O

Oberholzer, 91, 191
O'Gorman, 40, 186
Oppenheim, 137, 146, 197, 198
Orgler, 195
Ostertag, 148, 200

P

Parker, 196
Paskind, 112, 193
Patrick, 86, 190
Pearl, 78, 79, 188
Pearson, 87, 118, 142, 196
Penrose, 196
Peter, 22, 184
Pius XI, 60, 187
Plate, 188
Plesset, 160, 161, 202
Ploscowe, 151, 152, 202
Pollock, 27, 38, 42, 84, 86, 101, 104, 111, 186, 190, 192, 193
Popenoe, 5, 10, 41, 43, 46, 48, 117, 184, 186, 197, 203
Punnett, 64, 187

R

Reiter, 136, 196
Report of the Departmental Committee on Sterilization, His Majesty's Stationery Office, 21, 47, 65, 66, 67, 68, 119, 120, 184, 186
Riddle, 77, 188
Riebeth, 88, 190
Riedl, 151
Rife, 188
Riggenbach, 197
Roesle, 203
Rollin, 147
Rosanoff, 88, 91, 92, 118, 131, 159, 160, 161, 164, 167, 192, 196, 202
Rossman, J., 203
Rossman, M., 184
Rüdin, 25, 43, 53, 87, 91, 92, 93, 94, 95, 96, 97, 98, 107, 108, 151, 184, 186, 190, 192, 193, 202
Ruhemann, 148, 200
Ruttke, 184

S

Safran, 148, 200
Saleeby, 196
Schachter, 198
Schaffer, 147, 199
Schlub, 88
Schulz, 84, 101, 106, 107, 190, 192, 193
Schwesinger, 154, 196, 202
Shepardson, 146, 198
Sidler, 199
Siemens, 184
Sontag, 196
Spratling, 137
Stein, 85, 86, 139, 190, 197
Steuer, 201
Sticker, 151, 202
Stocks, 196
Stone, 197
Strauss, 148, 200
Struwe, 201
Stumpfl, 151, 202
Sünner, 192
Sydenstricker, 56

T

Taylor, 28, 30, 31, 32, 33, 185
Tenner, 148, 200
Terman, 170, 203
Thom, 138, 197
Timoféeff-Ressovsky, 75, 188
Tredgold, 55, 186, 196
Tucker, 147

U

Urechia, 198, 200
Usher, 196

V

von Verschuer, 156, 188, 202, 203
Vessie, 197
Vogt, 146, 188, 198

W

Wagner, 200
Wagner von Jauregg, 83, 190
Watkins, 184, 188
Weeks, 92, 197
Weinberg, 53, 91, 92, 93, 94, 96, 186, 192
Weitz, 199
Werthemann, 197
Whitney, 25, 59, 184, 187
Wilcox, 194
Wildenskov, 126, 196
Wilson, 196
Winston, 36, 37, 38, 186
Wittermann, 91, 92, 192
Woodall, 45, 186
Worster-Drought, 145, 147, 198, 199

Z

Zeleny, 188
Zurid, 201

SUBJECT INDEX

A

Accumulation rate of mental diseases, 26
Admission rates:
- and economic depression, 38
- and rural and urban environment, 27
- and social care, 27
- of Australia, 36
- of England and Wales, 36
- of Germany, 36
- of Massachusetts, 28
- of New York, 28
- of New Zealand, 36
- of Norway and Scandinavian countries, 36
- of Scotland, 36

Alcoholic psychoses:
- admission rates of, 29
- and schizophrenia, 97
- descendants of, 87
- marriage rates of, 41

Amaurotic idiocy:
- and sterilization, 180
- heredity of, 114

B

Birth rate of defective and insane groups, 25, 43, 44, 45, 46
Blastophoria, 3, 75

C

Castration:
- psychological nature of, 1

Chronic progressive neurological diseases:
- and sterilization, 180
- athetosis, 146
- chorea, 146
- diseases of peripheral nerves, 149
- Friedereich's ataxia, 146
- hereditary optic atrophy, 149
- Huntington's disease, 145, 179
- infantile diplegia and monoplegia, 148
- muscular dystrophy, 147
- myotonia, 147
- paroxysmal paralysis, 148
- progressive muscular atrophy, 147
- spastic spinal paralysis, 147
- syringomyelia, 148

Constitution, 75
Cretinism:
- heredity of, 112

Crime:
- conclusions on, 152
- definition of, 149
- identical twins and, 149, 166

Cultural compulsive (Calverton), 2

D

Death rate and mental disease, 51
Dementia praecox (see schizophrenia)
Diagnostic difficulties, 81
Divorce rate and mental diseases, 48

E

Economic depression and admission rate, 38
Epilepsy:
- and relation to first-born, 139
- and relation to feeblemindedness, 142
- and sterilization, 179
- and twins, 165
- conclusion of Committee on, 143
- death rate, 53
- heredity of, 84, 85, 99
  - early work on heredity of, 136
  - Mendelian nature of, 137
- incidence of, 141
- marriage rate, 41

Eugenics:
- and genius, 170
- origin of term, 2

Euthenics and natural selection, 25

F

Feebleminded and mentally deficient:
and genius, 171
and relation to epilepsy, 142
and sterilization, 179
and twins, 163
cerebral trauma and, 132
classification of, 112
conclusion of Committee on, 129
death rate, 53
heredity of, 114
Report of British Commission on, 119
community feebleminded, 123
institutional feebleminded, 123
marriage rate of, 41, 42, 45
Nams, Kallikaks, Jukes, etc., 47, 117
physical inferiority of, 124
premature birth and, 132
size of family and heredity of, 127

G

General paresis:
admission rate of, 29
marriage rate of, 41
Genetics:
and constitution, 78
and environment, 72
and experimental results, 77
and sterilization, 177
intra-genetic environment, 73
quantitativeness of gene, 75
Genius and sterilization, 170
and feebleminded, 171
and manic-depressive, 171
Gifted children, 170

H

Heredity:
and genius, 170
and sterilization, 178
normal and abnormal, 84, 99
Human Betterment Foundation, 10
Hydrocephalus:
heredity of, 114

I

Increase, alleged, of mental diseases, 24
Intelligence and environment:
experiments with foster children, 133
identical twins, 131, 155
influence of home, 134
relation of, 131

L

Laws concerning sterilization:
American and Canadian, 7
Foreign countries, 21

M

Manic-depressive psychosis:
admission rate of, 29
and genius, 171, 180
and sterilization, 179
and twins, 162
conclusions of Committee on, 110
death rate of, 53
distribution in average population, 107
heredity of, 99, 110
Marriage and mental disease, 41, 42, 43, 48, 56, 57, 183
Microcephalus:
heredity of, 114
Migraine:
heredity of, 85
Mongolism:
and twins, 164
heredity of, 113

O

Organic brain disease type of feeblemindedness:
and feeblemindedness, 132
heredity of, 113

P

Points of view regarding sterilization:
American Association for the Study of the Feebleminded, 68
British Commission, 65
Catholic, 61
eugenic, 59
genetic, 68
"ideal," 59
sociological, 64
Polymorphism:
criticism of, 83
theory of, 81
Population:
increasing age of, 34
Propagation rate of mentally diseased and defective, 40

R

Research and sterilization, 181

S

Schizophrenia (or dementia praecox):
  admission rate of, 29
  allelomorphic theory of, 91
  and alcoholism, 97
  and sterilization, 177, 180
  and twins, 158
  death rate of, 53
  descendants of, 87
  heredity of, 90, 99
    conclusion on, 107
  marriage rate of, 41
  occurrence in average population, 101
Selective sterilization, 16, 178
Senile psychoses:
  admission rate of, 29
Statistical method of Weinberg, 92
Sterilization:
  definition of, 4
  history of, 4
Subcultural groups, 114
Survival of fit, 2

T

Twins:
  and psychoses, 156
  conclusions of Committee on, 166
  identical, 131
    and crime, 149
  intelligence and, 155
  resemblance of, 153
  types of, 153

HISTORICAL ISSUES IN MENTAL HEALTH

An Arno Press Collection

American Psychopathological Association. **Trends Of Mental Disease.** 1945

Belknap, Ivan. **Human Problems Of A State Mental Hospital.** 1956

Berkley, Henry J. **A Treatise On Mental Diseases.** 1900

Bond, Earl D. **Thomas W. Salmon: Psychiatrist.** 1950

Briggs, L. Vernon. **Two Years' Service On The Reorganized State Board Of Insanity In Massachusetts,** August, 1914 to August, 1916. 1930

Briggs, L. Vernon. **A Victory For Progress In Mental Medicine.** 1924

Burrow, Trigant. **A Search For Man's Sanity.** 1958

Cahow, Clark R. **People, Patients and Politics.** (Doctoral Dissertation, Duke University, 1967). 1979

The Committee of the American Neurological Association for the Investigation of Eugenical Sterilization. **Eugenical Sterilization.** 1936

Cotton, Henry A. **The Defective Delinquent And Insane.** 1921

Dayton, Neil A. **New Facts On Mental Disorders.** 1940

Fein, Rashi. **Economics of Mental Illness.** 1958

Goldhamer, Herbert and Andrew W. Marshall. **Psychosis And Civilization.** 1953

Gosney, E.S., and Paul Popenoe. **Sterilization For Human Betterment.** 1929

Greenblat, Milton, et al. **From Custodial To Therapeutic Patient Care In Mental Hospitals.** 1955

Grob, Gerald N., editor. **Immigrants And Insanity.** 1979

Grob, Gerald N., editor. **Mental Hygiene In Twentieth Century America.** 1979

Grob, Gerald N., editor. **The Mentally Ill In Urban America.** 1979

Grob, Gerald N., editor. **The National Association For The Protection of the Insane And The Prevention Of Insanity.** 1979

Grob, Gerald N., editor. **Psychiatric Research In America.** 1979

Grob, Gerald N., editor. **Psychiatry and Medical Education.** 1979

Grob, Gerald N., editor. **Public Policy And Mental Illness.** 1979

Grimes, John Maurice. **Institutional Care Of Mental Patients In The United States.** 1934

Gurin, Gerald, et al. **Americans View Their Mental Health.** 1960

Hinsie, Leland. **The Treatment Of Schizophrenia.** 1930

Jahoda, Marie. **Current Concepts Of Positive Mental Health.** 1958

Joint Commission On Mental Illness And Health. **Action For Mental Health.** 1961

Koren, John. **Summaries Of State Laws Relating To The Insane.** 1917

Landis, Carney, and James D. Page. **Modern Society and Mental Disease.** 1938

Lewis, Nolan D.C. **Research In Dementia Praecox.** 1936

Malzberg, Benjamin. **Social And Biological Aspects Of Mental Disease.** 1940

May, James V. **Mental Diseases.** 1922

Myerson, Abraham. **Speaking Of Man.** 1950

The National Committee for Mental Hygiene. **State Hospitals In The Depression.** 1934

National Research Council, The Committee on Psychiatric Investigations. **The Problem Of Mental Disorder.** 1934

Plunkett, Richard J. and John E. Gordon,. **Epidemiology And Mental Illness.** 1960

Rapoport, Robert N., et al. **Community As Doctor.** 1960

Robison, Dale W. **Wisconsin And The Mentally Ill.** (Doctoral Dissertation, Marquette University, 1967). 1979

Sicherman, Barbara. **The Quest For Mental Health In America**, 1880-1917. (Doctoral Dissertation, Columbia University, 1967). 1979

Smith, Stephen. **Who Is Insane?** 1916

Stearns, Henry Putnam. **Insanity.** 1883

United States Surgeon General's Office. **The Medical Department Of The United States Army In The World War.** 1929

Wertheimer, F.I., and Florence E. Hesketh. **The Significance Of The Physical Constitution In Mental Disease.** 1926

White, William A. **The Mental Hygiene Of Childhood.** 1919

White, William A. **William Alanson White.** 1938